P9-BXY-148

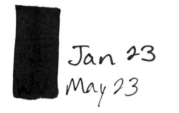
Jan 23
May 23

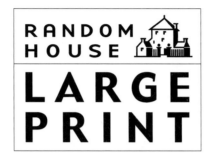

RANDOM
HOUSE

LARGE
PRINT

Also by Arthur Agatston, M.D.
available from Random House Large Print

The South Beach Diet
The South Beach Diet Cookbook

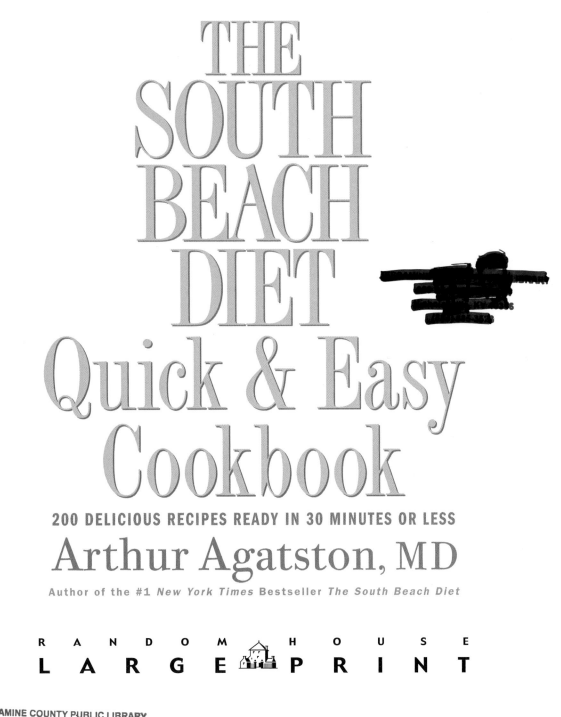

THE SOUTH BEACH DIET

Quick & Easy Cookbook

200 DELICIOUS RECIPES READY IN 30 MINUTES OR LESS

Arthur Agatston, MD

Author of the #1 *New York Times* Bestseller *The South Beach Diet*

RANDOM HOUSE
LARGE PRINT

Copyright © 2005 by Arthur Agatston, M.D.

Photographs © by Rodale Inc.

All rights reserved.
Published in the United States of America by
Random House Large Print in association with Rodale, New York.
Distributed by Random House, Inc., New York.

Book design by Carol Angstadt
Photography by Mitch Mandel
Food styling by Diane Simone Vezza
Prop styling by Melissa DeMayo

**The Library of Congress has established a
Cataloging-in-Publication record for this title.**

ISBN-13: 978-0-7393-2561-2
ISBN-10: 0-7393-2561-2

www.randomlargeprint.com

FIRST LARGE PRINT EDITION

10 9 8 7 6 5 4 3 2 1

This Large Print edition published in accord with the standards of the N.A.V.H.

To our mothers, Adell Agatston and Selma Fisher,

for their wonderful love and support over so many years.

And to my wife, Sari, for her continued love and support.

CONTENTS

ACKNOWLEDGMENTS

Since the publication of the first South Beach Diet book, Rodale has been a terrific home for us. I would like to thank Steve Murphy, Tami Booth Corwin, and Cindy Ratzlaff for their support, and my literary agent, Richard Pine, who brought us all together.

Thanks to everyone who contributed to this book, especially Carol Angstadt, art director **extraordinaire**, Nancy N. Bailey, JoAnn Brader, Mitch Mandel, and Diane Vezza. Special acknowledgments to Mindy Fox, who did a truly great job spearheading the recipe development for this project.

Many people are now involved with the South Beach Diet, and I want to thank all of our partners and members of the "brain trust" for sharing our vision and supporting the goal of changing the way America eats. And thanks to Ariel Rodriquez, my executive assistant, for keeping us all on track.

Special thanks to my sons, Evan and Adam, who are sources of frequent advice, whether I want it or not. I want to give **extra** special thanks to three fabulous women, without whom this book could not have been written. Margot Schupf, my editor, has become a great friend and advisor whose excellent judgment and dedication to this project have been invaluable. As I've often stated, I'm not a diet doctor, but with the help of my fantastic nutrition director, Marie Almon, I don't have to be. Her knowledge and hard work have been critical to the production of this book. Finally, thank you to my CEO, my best friend, my main advisor, and my partner—who also happens to be my wife, Sari. Her commitment to our common goals multiplies my productivity many times.

INTRODUCTION

For everyone who has struggled with weight loss and related health issues in the past, I have great news: The diet debates are over! After decades of confusing messages—"low fat" one day, "low carb" the next day, and "cabbage soup" the day after that (the medical community was just as confused as the public), we have actually achieved a consensus of opinion regarding the principles of healthy eating. Experts agree that we should be consuming the "right fats," the "right carbohydrates," "lean sources of protein," and "plenty of fiber." These are the principles of the South Beach Diet, and they have been successfully used for weight loss and better health by millions of people around the world.

If you're already a follower of the South Beach Diet, you know the facts: The "right fats" are the Mediterranean oils including olive oil, canola oil, flaxseed oil, and omega-3 fish oil, as well as the fats found in most nuts. The "right carbohydrates" are the nutrient- and fiber-rich vegetables, whole fruits, and whole grains. Lean sources of protein include fish, chicken, and lean cuts of meats, as well as low-fat dairy and plant sources such as beans and soy. Our good sources of fiber come from consuming enough of the right carbs.

If the diet debates are over, then the challenge becomes how to incorporate these universally accepted principles into our everyday eating habits. I've learned from experience that dieters who have the most success are the ones who enjoy a wide variety of foods and diverse ways to prepare them. But we all share the burden of today's fast-paced society, when time is our most valuable commodity (after health) and other things are sacrificed. So many people loved our first South Beach Diet cookbook but said they didn't always have time to prepare the recipes—they wanted more recipes that could be prepared quickly and easily. This new **South Beach Diet Quick & Easy Cookbook** is our answer to those requests, and it's designed to help you make this way of eating a way of life!

The Roots of Modern Eating Habits

For us to better understand what's changed in the American diet over the past 40 years and why those changes have led to our current epidemic of obesity and disease, it's helpful to start at the beginning. Really, the very beginning: the beginning of human existence on earth. Believe it or not, early man's eating and exercise habits determined what our healthy eating and exercise habits should be today.

Man lived for thousands of years wandering the earth in small tribes. Because of their lifestyle, these people were referred to as "hunter-gatherers." What they hunted were game animals that grazed on grasses and were comprised of lean meat and (unlike grain-fed cattle and poultry) good fats. What they gathered were whole fruits and vegetables. All this hunting and gathering took a lot of energy and exertion, making regular exercise an integral part of their daily life.

Life for hunter-gatherers was difficult. It's not like they could open the refrigerator and get something to eat. But interestingly, they were drawn to specific foods—sweet, salty, and/or fatty—whose nutritional properties enabled them to survive. The available sweet foods were fruits and vegetables. Sweet berries are loaded with essential vitamins, nutrients (including antioxidants), and fiber. The salt in salty foods helps to maintain blood volume and is also essential for cells to function. Their attraction to fat led them to hunting big game, which were fattier than small game and were good sources of protien. Fat helps store energy as well as maintain important bodily structures and functions, such as the nervous system.

Our ancestors' craving for foods that were sweet, salty, and fatty drew them to foods that were essential for their health. And since there was no way to procure those foods other than hunting and gathering, for early man, they were the equivalent of fast foods. If you think about it, these patterns of being attracted to sweet, salty, and fatty foods are still the prevalent patterns in how we eat today. So our fast-paced lives are not the only reason we choose fast foods: Our natural taste buds that helped us survive in a "natural" environment now lead us to the worst food choices in today's very "unnatural" surroundings.

There is more to learn from early man that explains other of our modern health problems. Right now, 40 percent of Americans between the ages of 40 and 70 are prediabetic and 70 percent or more of those in cardiac-care units are found to be diabetic or prediabetic. What's the connection to early man here?

Type 2, or so-called "adult onset" diabetes (which unfortunately is now found in adolescents and even preadolescent children) occurs when the pancreas gradually "burns out." It essentially gets tired of producing the excess insulin required to contend with the unprecedented amounts of sugar and starch (in the form of processed carbohydrates) in the American diet. This means that when sugar and fats flood our bloodstream after a meal, there is insufficient insulin to efficiently move these nutrients into our tissues for immediate fuel or for storage.

Another factor that stresses our pancreatic reserves is "insulin resistance." As we gain weight in our bellies and our fat cells get bigger, a "resistance" to the action of insulin occurs. It takes greater quantities of insulin to move sugar and fat into our tissues. This results in higher insulin levels and a greater strain on our pancreas. This, in turn, raises our levels of blood sugar while the insulin is trying to work, which then leads to a more rapid and deeper drop in our blood sugar levels when the insulin finally does unlock our tissues to allow for absorption of blood sugar. This drop in blood sugar is known as "reactive hypoglycemia" and is responsible for severe food cravings in those with insulin resistance or prediabetes. Our actual insulin levels are elevated in this condition, just not high enough to do the job.

So what does the life of early man have to do with this phenomenon? Insulin resistance and the resulting exaggerated swings in blood sugar was actually a survival mechanism for early man, who regularly contended with cycles of feast and famine. During times of feast, when food was plentiful—often the summer and fall—man was hungrier and ate more, and fuel in the form of belly fat could be stored. When food was scarce or famine arrived—often in winter months—then man could live off the stored fat and would be more likely to survive. So when food was available, man was able to store fat, his fat cells got bigger, causing insulin resistance, and that resulted in great swings in blood sugar, more hunger, and more fuel/fat storage. The fat storage enabled man to survive the oncoming period of famine. In science, this is actually known as the "thrifty gene theory." It is interesting to note that societies such as the Pima Indians, who have experienced subsistence living (like the hunter-gatherers) in recent generations, have a particularly strong dose of this genetic predisposition and also have epidemic levels of obesity and diabetes when exposed to a Western diet. For modern Americans living without times of famine, the increased hunger associated with insulin resistance just makes us fatter and fatter. When our pancreases tire of producing so much insulin, we also become diabetic.

There's another phenomenon of modern life, "yo-yo dieting," that can also be better understood from the perspective of the early man's survival. Let's return to the challenge of living through famine. When food was scarce and caloric intake quickly became severely restricted, it was helpful that rapid weight loss was associated with a slowing of our metabolism. We could then live on fewer calories and be more likely to survive. This still happens now. When we lose weight rapidly by either naturally imposed or voluntary caloric restriction, we lose not just fat but also muscle. Muscle is more metabolically active than fat even at rest, so that when we lose it, our metabolism slows and we require fewer calories to live. This meant a better chance of survival for early man experiencing famine. For modern dieters who decide rapid weight loss is desirable, it means a slowed metabolism just like for early man. But for the majority of us, it begins the cycle of yo-yo dieting. Fewer calories are required to maintain our weight, and it becomes harder and harder to continue to lose. This invariably leads to regaining the lost weight, and then some. This is why quick-weight-loss plans don't have lasting effects and are really counterproductive in the end.

A Nation of Fast Food

Let's apply what we learned from early man's survival to our present situation. We'll jump ahead from the time of the hunter-gatherer to the United States after World War II. In the 1950s and 1960s, the food intake of populations around the world was studied in an attempt to explain America's

relatively high rates of heart attacks and strokes. These studies indicated that in societies following a low-fat, high-carbohydrate diet (at that time, the less developed countries), heart attacks and strokes as well as obesity were rare occurrences. In high-fat, low-carbohydrate consuming societies (northern Europe and the United States), heart attacks and strokes were common. So in the 1960s, it seemed logical to put Americans on a low-fat, high-carb diet to curb our growing rate of heart disease. This was done and was reflected in the national guidelines that began to emerge in the late 1960s and later morphed into the USDA food pyramid. These guidelines were based on consumption of cereals, bread, and rice, with fats to be consumed in very limited amounts.

The national recommendations led to an experiment with unintended results. Rather than becoming thinner and healthier, we became fatter and sicker. The prevalence of obesity and diabetes soared, and 45 years later it's affecting not only the adult population but also our teens and preteens. Some believe the present generation of young Americans will be the first to have a shorter life expectancy than their parents.

To see how this relates to our present obesity crisis, we need to examine the problems with the science that led to the national recommendations. Looking back at the original studies done in the 1950s and 1960s, we realize now that the traditional carbohydrates consumed by the less-developed countries who followed the low-fat, high-carbohydrate diet were unprocessed, high in fiber, and high in nutrient value and had low glycemic indices, which meant they were slowly digested. What the American food industry introduced in response to the guidelines and the resulting consumer demand were processed carbohydrates where the fiber and its associated nutrients were removed. The reason? At that time, we did not understand the role of fiber in our digestive process or the strong association between fiber and essential nutrients. We also did not understand how digested carbohydrates contributed to the exaggerated swings in blood sugar associated with obesity, prediabetes, and diabetes.

Other phenomena occurring during this period were longer workdays at more sedentary jobs and our ever-increasing lack of time. The traditional family sit-down dinner made with whole foods that took hours to prepare became largely a thing of the past. The demand for fast, convenient foods grew, and the food and restaurant industry responded. Remember that if we just follow our hunter-gatherer taste buds, we will be drawn directly to sweet, salty, and fatty fast foods.

The result of all these factors? We became the first fast-food nation in the history of the world. We consumed rapidly digested foods devoid of fiber and nutrients, and we consumed them rapidly, often eating on the run instead of taking the time to savor the meal. Less apparent than our increasing waistlines is the fact that while we are **overfed,** we are **undernourished**—literally malnourished due to the absence of nutrients in our fast, convenient foods. This type of malnutrition is especially prevalent in our children. Often they are on a nearly pure starch and sugar diet lacking vitamins, minerals, and nutrients. I believe that much of what we label as attention deficit syndrome leading to academic and behavior problems are diet-related. For adults, our poor nutrition appears to contribute not just to obesity and diabetes but also to cancer, arthritis, Alzheimer's disease, and many other chronic illnesses.

So we now know how we need to eat. We must follow the principles of good fats, good carbs, lean sources of protein, and plenty of fiber. How do we do it? We stock our kitchens with good foods and make the right choices. In this book, you'll find 200 wonderful recipes that can be prepared with readily available ingredients, most of which are ready in 30 minutes or less.

This **South Beach Diet Quick & Easy Cookbook** is meant to be one small step in our strategy to make healthy eating easier for the modern "fast family." Incorporating the principles outlined will pay dividends, not just in reducing our waistlines but also in our general health. So take a lesson from the Boy Scouts and be prepared. If you keep your kitchen stocked and these recipes on hand, you'll be well on your way to good health.

HOW TO MAKE THE SOUTH BEACH DIET QUICK AND EASY

This cookbook offers many easy and delicious foods that you can enjoy while you lose weight and improve your overall health. As you eat better, you'll not only look and feel better but also improve your blood chemistry and reduce your risk for prediabetes and a host of other diseases.

If you're already familiar with the South Beach Diet, you'll know that it's divided into three phases. Phase 1, which lasts for the first two weeks, will help you kick-start your weight loss while you learn what foods to enjoy and which to avoid. You'll be losing weight and improving your blood chemistry by ending the cycle of insulin resistance associated with cravings. While you eat plenty of lean protein, veggies, nuts, reduced-fat cheese, eggs, and low-fat dairy, you'll cut out all starches, including pasta, rice, and bread. You'll also eliminate sugar, which includes all fruits and juices. You'll eat three meals a day plus two snacks, and even a dessert snack.

In Phase 2, your cravings will have subsided, and you'll

continue to lose weight at a steady rate. You'll gradually add more of the right carbs—including whole-grain breads, whole-wheat pasta, and brown rice—back into your diet, and you'll reintroduce fruits and some root vegetables that were off-limits during Phase 1. You'll start to reintroduce these foods slowly and see how much you can enjoy while continuing to lose weight. Note that you can also start the diet in Phase 2 if you don't have much weight to lose (generally 10 pounds or less and don't have a significant problem with cravings) or are following this plan primarily for health rather than weight-loss reasons. Remember that even if you don't have any weight to lose, following the principles of the South Beach Diet is still the healthiest way to eat.

Finally, once you reach a healthy weight for you, you'll enter Phase 3. At this point, you'll know what you can eat while maintaining your health and your weight. Since there is no list of forbidden foods in Phase 3, you'll have more latitude when it comes to enjoying occasional items you were not allowing yourself in Phase 2. As long as you stick to the principles of your South Beach lifestyle and remember to monitor how your particular body responds to the foods you are eating, you'll continue to improve your health and maintain your weight, while enjoying a host of wonderful foods and a way of life that has now become second nature.

If you're looking after your family's health as well as your own, you're in luck. Kids will love the home-cooked meals you'll make from this book. Dishes like Baked Barbecue Chicken (page 308), Pork Fajitas (page 312), the South Beach Classic Burger (page 316), South Beach Macaroni and Cheese (page 376), and Tempeh Tacos (page 394) will appeal to the whole family. It is important that they learn the principles of good eating as early as possible.

I know how easy it is to resort to convenient drive-through restaurants, especially when time is limited. So I've included many recipes throughout this book that take less than 15 minutes to prepare, plus quick-cook ideas that don't even require a formal recipe (see page 58). In the same amount of time that it takes to pick up an order at a fast-food restaurant, you'll be able to prepare delicious, healthy meals. You'll see that it is possible to have a "fast-food" lifestyle that is also nutritious. In fact, the meals in this cookbook are so flavorful that your family may not even realize that they are also good for them!

How This Book Is Organized

If you're a busy person who loves food but doesn't have a lot of time to cook, this book is for you. Designed to save you both shopping and cooking time, the majority of dishes in the book require just 10 ingredients or less and take less than 30 minutes to cook. As in the *South Beach Diet Cookbook,* chapters are arranged by type of meal or central ingredient; you'll find everything from savory breakfast and brunch dishes to scrumptious soups, snacks, and salads; fantastic fish, chicken, and meat entrées; and delectable desserts.

Phase 1, 2, and 3 designations are clear, so you can add new recipes to your repertoire as you reach your desired goals. Remember that once you move into later phases, when the South Beach Diet has become a lifestyle, you can still go back and enjoy your favorite meals from earlier phases. And as with all South Beach recipes, no matter what phase you're in, you'll find that the portions are ample and the ideas are exciting and fresh.

You'll notice that each recipe in this book includes prep and cook times, so you can plan your time accordingly. On those days when you want to fit in a class at the gym or run an extra errand, you'll probably turn to a recipe that takes 15 minutes or less from start to finish (look for the icon that denotes a "superfast" recipe). When you have a little extra time to prepare a meal, you may choose a recipe that requires a 20- or 30-minute cook time.

We've included just a few recipes that are just as simple as the others but may require a 30- to 40-minute cook time. We felt they were too good to leave out! If the recipe does take more than 30 minutes, you'll see a note in the introduction explaining why it's well worth devoting a little extra time to achieve the wonderful results you'll get.

It is my hope that by having the approximate times you'll need for each recipe, you'll have a multitude of great choices that work well with your schedule on any given day. And to make things even easier, I've provided Quick Tips and Smart Cook suggestions throughout this chapter, plus a special section on getting ahead (see page 65) so that when you're ready to prepare meals, you can significantly reduce your prep time.

If the key to achieving your goals is simple, fast, and tasty meals, I feel confident that you'll find success (and plenty of delectable dishes that will easily fit into your lifestyle) in the pages of this book.

South Beach Diet Quick and Easy Kitchen

Time and time again, I notice that the people who struggle most with a healthy eating plan are those who haven't organized in advance. If you arrive home from a busy day at work and your cupboards are bare, you're more likely to call out for a pizza or hit a drive-through on the way home. If you have unhealthy snack foods lying around the kitchen (like cookies, candy, snack cakes, potato chips, and sugared sodas), you're more apt to consume them instead of enjoying nutrient-dense foods, like nuts, low-fat cheeses, and fiber-rich fruits that are healthier than commercial snack foods and will satisfy you longer.

The same goes for quick lunches. Putting together meals to take with you to the office or to school helps you resist the urge to eat processed convenience foods and vending machine snacks. Best of all, since you've prepared your lunch in advance, no matter how busy you become during the day, you can rest assured that a nutritious, energy-replenishing meal awaits you.

So how do you get organized? You'll begin by clearing the "bad" foods from your kitchen and replenishing your cupboards and fridge with "good" South Beach-friendly items. In the pages that follow, you'll find a glossary of essential ingredients you'll soon become familiar with, if you're not already. We've put these items into an alphabetical format so that you can find helpful information fast when you're unfamiliar with an ingredient or when you want to know more about its health benefits.

South Beach Quick and Easy Essentials

With these essential ingredients on hand, you'll be able to put together a quick and easy South Beach meal anytime. Use this glossary both as an informative guide and as a shopping checklist, to help you to keep your pantry, fridge, and freezer stocked with good staples.

With the exception of cereals, grains, pastas, and fruits (which are reintroduced in Phase 2), most of these ingredients are fine for any phase of the South Beach Diet. Though the majority of these items can be found in most supermarkets, we've clearly marked specialty store or Internet purchase items so that you'll be able to easily find them, too.

Glossary of Ingredients

Throughout the glossary, we point out convenience products that will help speed up your prep times, allowing you to put a meal on the table in, sometimes, just minutes. Note that these items (such as packaged washed and torn lettuces or cooked chicken strips) will surely save you time, but depending on the ingredient, they may be more costly than ingredients that require preparation at home. If the convenience is worth a little more to you at the checkout line, go for it. If not, that's okay, too—all you'll add to your time in the kitchen is a few more minutes.

APPLES: Providing both insoluble and soluble fiber (known to be helpful in lowering cholesterol levels), apples also offer vitamin C and potassium. A few slices make a great snack, but you can also enjoy apples in savory dishes like Apple-Butternut Squash Soup (page 125) and Rosemary Pork Medallions with Chunky Applesauce (page 314). To pick the best, look for firm to hard specimens with unbroken skins.

QUICK TIP: To prevent apple slices as well as fresh artichokes from browning while preparing a dish, drop them into a bowl filled with cold water and a good squeeze of fresh lemon juice.

APRICOTS: These soft-fleshed fruits are a good source of vitamins A and C, fiber, potassium, and iron. They are available fresh in late spring and summer and dried year-round; use them to gently sweeten our heart-healthy Spiced Oatmeal with Dried Apricot and Walnuts (page 88).

ARTICHOKES: An excellent source of fiber, artichokes also provide vitamin C, iron, potassium, magnesium, and folate. Fresh artichokes are available in the springtime in both large and "baby" sizes. For quick and easy recipes, you're more likely to rely on the convenient frozen, canned, or jarred varieties or the marinated artichokes from the deli case. They'll help you make dishes like Sirloin Steak with Artichokes, Tomatoes, and Olives (page 331) and Warm Artichoke Dip (page 147). Rinse brine-packed artichokes before using if you're concerned about your sodium intake.

ARUGULA: An Italian salad green with a delightfully peppery flavor, arugula is delicious in salads (on its own or mixed with other greens), sandwiches, and pasta dishes.

ASPARAGUS: A fiber-rich source of beta-carotene, vitamin C, and iron, asparagus is available fresh in the spring and canned or frozen year-round. Use it as a side dish or chopped up in pastas and salads.

QUICK TIP: Roll up a piece of blanched or grilled asparagus in a slice of roast beef or smoked salmon for a delicious and healthy snack.

AVOCADO: Mild and delicious with a smooth, buttery texture, avocados are a favorite in salads, sandwiches, and quesadillas. You might also enjoy them in place of butter as a spread for whole-grain crackers or bread. Avocados provide vitamin C and folate. Their fat is mostly monounsaturated, which is helpful in lowering LDL cholesterol levels, but because they are high in calories, you'll want to limit your daily intake to about one-quarter of a whole avocado. A ripe avocado will yield to your gentle pressing.

QUICK TIP: To ripen an unripe avocado, place it in a brown paper bag and leave it at room temperature for 2 to 4 days. Be sure to check frequently so you don't overripen the fruit.

BABA GHANOUSH: This tasty Middle Eastern purée is made from cooked eggplant, tahini, olive oil, and lemon juice. It makes a wonderful dip for fresh vegetables. You can also use it as a sandwich filling or spread. Prepared baba ghanoush is readily available in most supermarkets.

BACON: Go for turkey or Canadian bacon; both have the same smoky taste you love from regular bacon, with less saturated fat than the regular kind.

BANANAS: High in vitamin B_6, bananas also provide pectin, a soluble fiber that helps lower cholesterol levels. An occasional banana (choose a medium one) makes a good snack. For dessert, try our heavenly Mexican-Style Chocolate Bananas (page 444).

BARLEY: This nutritious grain provides protein as well as ample B vitamins, iron, zinc, and selenium (an antioxidant). Quick-cooking (or instant) barley contains the same nutrients as the regular kind and cuts cooking time from about 45 minutes to just 10. You can use barley in salads or in place of whole-grain brown rice in stuffed peppers or pilafs.

BEANS AND LEGUMES: A fantastic source of protein and fiber, beans are helpful in the control of diabetes because the body digests them slowly, allowing a gradual release of blood glucose. Delicious in soups, stews, and salads, most beans and legumes are widely available both canned and dried. The canned varieties are among the most convenient products when it comes to quickly preparing tasty soups, stews, and salads. Dried legumes (e.g., lentils) and beans (including chickpeas) should be stored in a cool, dry place for no longer than 1 year; soak dried beans for 12 hours before cooking.

QUICK TIP: To keep cook times short for dried beans, try to get relatively fresh ones. Look for sell-by dates on packages of dried beans and legumes or purchase them from a reputable grocer with high turnover. If packages don't have dates, use a permanent marker to mark them yourself with the purchase date. Though they will not go bad, as they age, dried beans and legumes become less fresh and actually take longer to cook!

Here are a few of the beans that are used in this book.

• **Black beans:** Native to South America and used heavily in Mexican and Latin American cooking, black beans are also known as Mexican, Spanish, or black turtle beans. An excellent source of iron, magnesium, phosphorus, and folate, black beans make great additions to salads and burritos. Try them in the Chipotle Beef Burrito (page 368) or served with whole-grain brown rice and no-sugar-added salsa.

• **Black soybeans:** These beans are just as delicious as regular black beans, yet they're higher in protein, fiber, and potassium. Soybeans are also the only beans that provide complete protein, making their protein comparable to dairy protein. Look for canned black soybeans in health food stores and try them in any recipe that calls for black beans. You may find you need to add seasoning as black soybeans tend to have a less rich flavor than regular black beans. If a recipe calls for black soybeans and they aren't available, use regular black beans.

• **Cannellini beans:** These white Italian beans (also called white kidney beans) have a nutty flavor and creamy texture. You'll love them in bean salads, minestrone soups, and our Turkey and White Bean Chili (page 293).

• **Chickpeas (or garbanzo beans):** A favorite ingredient in the Mediterranean, India, and the Middle East, these delicious legumes have a mild nutty flavor and a firm yet creamy texture. Packed with protein, fiber, good carbs, folate, iron, and zinc, they're perfect for soups, stews, pastas, and salads. Try them in our Turkey Sausages with Kale and Chickpeas (page 272) and Tofu, Chickpea, and Sun-Dried Tomato Salad (page 378).

• **Edamame:** These fresh soybeans are a boon for quick and easy recipes. They come shelled and frozen, making it easy to drop a handful into soups, salads, and bean purées. Like black soybeans (see above), they provide a complete protein, and they're delicious. Give them a try in Gingered Tofu Salad (page 383) and Soupe au Pistou (page 385).

• **Lentils:** Mild in flavor and high in protein and fiber, these small, round seeds are native to southwestern Asia. You may also see them labeled as green lentils, Egyptian lentils, German lentils, and Indian brown lentils. They're tasty in soups, stews, and salads.

• **Pinto beans:** Also known as red Mexican beans, pintos are named for their pinkish-brown streaks (*pinto* is Spanish for "painted"), which disappear when the beans are cooked. You'll often find them in chili, but they can also be used in soups, salads, tacos, and more.

• **Soybeans:** See Edamame, above, and Black soybeans on page 10.

• **Split peas:** These nutty-tasting legumes are highly nutritious. Even in their dried form they do not require soaking, and they cook quickly. Use them to make your own split pea soup. You can also purchase canned split peas.

SMART COOK: To get a full set of essential amino acids, combine any kind of bean with grains in soups, salads, or even burritos (see our Veggie Burrito, page 380).

BEEF: A great source of iron, zinc, vitamin B$_{12}$, and protein, beef is also delicious and easy to cook. And since Americans began demanding leaner meats over the last decade or so, cattle are now being bred to produce leaner, lower-fat meats. Still, not all cuts of beef are created equal when it comes to fat. Look for lean cuts like flank steak, London broil, tenderloin (filet mignon), T-bone, top round, bottom round, eye of round, sirloin, and top loin; veal chops and cutlets are also fine. Avoid porterhouse, rib roast, rib steaks, and brisket, which are high in fat. When choosing ground beef, look for extra lean, lean, or sirloin. Before cooking beef, trim the remaining visible fat.

BLACKBERRIES: A great source of the antioxidant vitamin C, blackberries also offer folate, iron, and pectin (a soluble fiber that may help to reduce cholesterol levels). Snack on these plump, tasty berries or use them in green or fruit salads.

BLUEBERRIES: Chock-full of disease-fighting antioxidants and fiber and a great source of vitamin C, fresh blueberries are available most of the year. Sweet and juicy, they're great mixed into low-fat or fat-free plain yogurt (an instant breakfast, snack, or dessert) and wonderful in our Blueberry Buckwheat Pancakes (page 82). Blueberries are also available frozen.

SMART COOK: When cooking or baking with frozen berries, use them in their frozen state (not thawed) and add them just before cooking to keep their juices from bleeding out.

SMART COOK: To keep berries fresh for as long as possible, don't wash them until you're ready to use them.

BRAN: A great source of fiber and magnesium, bran is the nutritious outer covering of wheat grain. Use it in our tasty Pear Bran Muffins (page 105).

BREAD: Choose 100 percent whole-grain bread (try multigrain, oat and bran, rye, sprouted grain, buckwheat, whole wheat, or other similar types) containing at least 3 grams of dietary fiber per slice for Phases 2 and 3. Bread is off-limits in Phase 1.

BREAD CRUMBS: Look for whole-wheat bread crumbs (Italian or plain) and store them in the freezer so they stay fresh over time. Bread crumbs are off-limits in Phase 1.

SMART COOK: Store sliced whole-grain bread in the freezer, where it will keep for months and a slice is always ready when you need one. No need to thaw frozen bread slices, just toast and use. This allows you to use just one or two slices at a time and not feel pressured to finish the whole bag before its sell-by date.

BROCCOLI: Another nutritional powerhouse, fiber-rich broccoli is packed with folate, riboflavin, potassium, iron, and vitamin C. Broccoli also supplies abundant amounts of cancer-fighting carotenoids and phytochemicals. You'll find broccoli in the produce section, where the florets also often come in packaged ready-to-cook broccoli and carrot mix, stir-fry mix, and vegetable medley; these are all acceptable in Phases 2 and 3 (when you can reintroduce carrots) for stir-frying, roasting, or steaming. Broccoli is also available frozen.

QUICK TIP: Packaged broccoli and cauliflower florets are available in the produce section of many supermarkets; they'll save you valuable trimming and cutting time.

BROWN RICE: This wholesome rice is rich in thiamin, niacin, vitamin B_6, and fiber; use it as a side dish, salad ingredient, or burrito filling. When it comes to saving time, parboiled or precooked brown rice is a lifesaver—just make sure to purchase brands that do not include partially hydrogenated oils. Uncle Ben's Natural Whole Grain Brown Rice and Kraft Minute Instant Whole Grain Brown Rice are both good bets. Avoid rice packaged in a pouch with seasoning.

BROTHS: High-quality chicken, beef, vegetable, and seafood broths are widely available, making it easy to make quick soups and stews at home. Be sure to purchase lower sodium varieties. Broths packaged in resealable boxes make it easy to refrigerate unused portions. You can also freeze cooled, unused portions in labeled plastic containers for future use; leave an inch or two of space in the container, as foods will expand as they freeze.

QUICK TIP: For an easy flavor boost, use lower sodium broths (any type) in place of or mixed with water to cook whole-wheat couscous, whole-grain brown rice, or grains— a great use for leftover broths.

BUCKWHEAT: A supplier of protein, B vitamins, potassium, iron, and calcium, buckwheat is neither a wheat nor a grain but actually an herb. Perfect for people who suffer from gluten intolerance or wheat allergies (and otherwise a delicious alternative to the usual grains for the rest of us), buckwheat comes in the form of flour, which you can use to make delicious pancakes (see Blueberry Buckwheat Pancakes on page 82), and in groats (see Kasha on page 35), which can be blended with or used in place of brown rice or grains. Buckwheat has a wonderfully toasty, nutty flavor. Look for buckwheat products in both supermarkets and health food stores.

BULGUR: This heart-healthy source of fiber, protein, B vitamins, iron, and magnesium is made from steamed, dried, cracked wheat berries. Often used in Mediterranean and Middle Eastern dishes—and best known for its use in the Middle Eastern salad tabbouli—bulgur has a light, nutty flavor. Try it in our tasty Eggplant Bulgur Lasagna (page 409).

BUTTER-FLAVORED FAT-FREE COOKING SPRAY: Use this to add a light butter flavor to foods while preventing them from sticking to the pan.

CABBAGE: A great supplier of potential cancer-fighting phytochemicals, this crunchy crucifer is also rich in vitamin C, fiber, and folate. Many supermarkets sell shredded cabbage, as well as cole slaw mix (which is mostly cabbage with some carrot) in ready-to-go packs in the pro-duce section. You can use this to whip up our South Beach Cole Slaw (page 438).

CANTALOUPE: High in vitamins A and C, beta-carotene, and potassium, cantaloupe is available in spring and summer. Though you'll often find cubed melon in supermarkets, it's best to buy a whole melon and cut it yourself, as exposure to oxygen will cause a decrease in the fruit's nutrients. In Phases 2 and 3, melons make a great breakfast, snack, or even dessert. For a refreshing treat on a hot night, try Melon Slush (page 479).

CAPERS: Tiny, tangy, and slightly salty, these sun-dried flower buds make delicious sauces for chicken, meat, fish, and pasta dishes (see Crispy Trout with Lemon-Caper Sauce, page 227). Found in the condiment section of most supermarkets, capers are packed in either salt or brine. Remember to rinse them with water before using to remove excess salt.

CARROTS: Available year-round, carrots are sweet-tasting and high in vitamin A. Reintroduce them to your diet in Phases 2 and 3. Try them steamed, sautéed with other veggies, or roughly chopped, drizzled with olive oil, and roasted.

CAULIFLOWER: A member of the cabbage family, cauliflower contains beneficial phytochemicals and also provides fiber, folate, and vitamin B_6. Cauliflower is often served steamed but is also remarkably delicious when roasted, sautéed, or puréed into a soup. Try Creamy Cauliflower Soup (page 118), Cauliflower and Kale Bake (page 390), and Roasted Spicy Cauliflower (page 415).

CELERY ROOT: A close relative of celery, celery root (or celeriac) is a round, knobby root vegetable with a tough skin. Use it as an incredibly flavorful addition to salads, soups, and stews. Cut celery root into thin matchsticks if eating it raw; peel, cube, and toss it with olive oil and salt and pepper and roast it until golden; or braise or boil it until tender. If you've never tried this tasty vegetable, our Celery Root and Turnip Mash (page 436) is a perfect place to start.

CHIPOTLES IN ADOBO: A favorite quick and easy ingredient, these smoked, dried jalapeño chiles come in cans and are packed in a dark red sauce made from vinegar and other seasonings. Both the peppers and the sauce add punch to chili and other dishes; use them in our Beef and Bean Chili (page 341) and in our vegetarian Quick Bean Chili (page 399).

CHARD (OR SWISS CHARD): This leafy cruciferous vegetable scores high in vitamins A and C and is also a great source of iron. Common varieties include ruby chard and rainbow chard. Discard chard's tough stems but thinly slice and steam or sauté the tender ones together with the leaves.

CHEESE: A great source of calcium and protein, cheese can be high in saturated fat and calories. Choose low- or reduced-fat varieties that contain no more than 6 grams of fat per serving. Cheeses are great for snacking as well as for cooking in casseroles, pastas, salads, sandwiches, sauces, and more.

The following types of cheeses are often used in South Beach recipes.

• **Cheddar cheese:** This firm cow's milk cheese is available in a range of flavors from mild to sharp. Use the reduced-fat variety.

• **Cream cheese:** Low- and reduced-fat varieties of cream cheese make great spreads as well as omelet and cheesecake fillings. Our Celery with Herbed Cream Cheese and Walnuts (page 141) makes a yummy snack or appetizer.

• **Feta:** Crumble this tangy Greek cheese into salads and over chicken dishes.

• **Goat cheese:** Goat cheese (or chèvre) has a creamy texture and tart flavor. Use it to liven up salads or as a spread for vegetables or whole-grain crackers or toast.

• **Laughing Cow Light:** Kids and adults alike love this creamy, smooth cow's milk cheese for its mild flavor and fun packaging. Its single-wrapped portions make an easy, fuss-free take-along snack on their own. Or enjoy them on whole-grain crackers, spread into celery sticks, or in sandwiches.

• **Monterey Jack:** This delicious, ivory-colored cow's milk cheese is great for melting and for sandwiches. Look for the reduced-fat version and try pepper Jack when you want an extra kick!

• **Mozzarella:** Delicious in salads, sandwiches, and pastas and great melted or at room temperature. Choose the skim-milk version.

• **Parmesan:** This nutty-tasting hard cheese is at its best when freshly grated. A small chunk will keep in your fridge for 2 weeks in a resealable bag (press the air out) in your produce compartment. Since Parmesan is so versatile, delicious, and full-flavored, we use it in many of our recipes. It does, however, have just over 8 grams of fat per ounce, so you'll want to use less than 1 ounce per serving (up to 3 tablespoons). A little goes a long way, in this case!

• **Provolone:** This Italian cow's milk cheese is great for melting.

• **Ricotta:** This smooth cheese resembles cottage cheese but is sweeter and, surprisingly, has four times more calcium. It's delicious in pastas (like our Whole-Wheat Penne with Eggplant and Ricotta, page 396) and desserts (like the popular Ricotta Crème, found in the original South Beach Diet book and on the South Beach Diet Web site). Look for part-skim ricotta, which has all the flavor of the whole-milk version but 40 percent less fat.

• **Swiss:** This favorite holey cheese is great for sandwiches and melted into egg dishes, like our Swiss Cheese and Vegetable Omelet (page 80). Look for the reduced-fat variety.

QUICK TIP: Look for shredded reduced- and low-fat cheeses in the dairy case at most supermarkets—they're ready to sprinkle onto salads, pastas, rice dishes, vegetables, eggs, and more and will help you save prep and cleanup time.

CHERRIES: A good cherry bursts with juicy flavor, and a handful of the fruit makes a refreshing, sweet snack. Cherries are a great source of vitamin C. Though fresh ones are only available in the summer months, you'll find frozen cherries (already pitted for you!) year-round—perfect for our Cherry Spoon Sweet with Yogurt (page 464).

CHILI PASTE: A spicy, red Asian condiment often flavored with garlic, chili paste is widely used in Chinese cooking. A great way to spice up a dish, it can be found in the Asian foods section of large supermarkets or in Asian markets. Use it in dishes like Thai Grilled Beef with String Beans (page 318) or even to spice up dishes like plain old chicken soup.

CHILE PEPPERS: These peppery favorites make great flavor boosters to all kinds of meat and vegetarian dishes. Look for the wide array of canned chiles that are available to help you make quick meals (see our Spiced Grouper with Mild Chile Purée, page 203). You might also want to try pickled jalapeños, which make a good snack if you like spicy foods; or you can chop and sprinkle them into burritos or salads and over tostadas.

CHOCOLATE: Unless you're just starting the South Beach Diet, you know that chocolate is allowed, but only in moderation. As you progress with the diet, it's okay to enjoy a small amount of dark chocolate. See the dessert chapter for innovative recipes that offer you just enough of the sweet treat per serving. And remember that it's important to stick to the recommended serving portions.

COCOA POWDER: Keep unsweetened cocoa powder on hand to make desserts like Green Tea Truffles (page 442) and Mini Cocoa Swirl Cheesecakes (page 445).

COCONUT MILK: Coconut milk is made from coconut and water steeped together to produce a coconut-flavored liquid that is a wonderful base for soup and rice dishes. It's widely used in Indian and Southeast Asian cooking (see Indian Chicken, page 254, and Chicken Green Curry, page 304). You'll want to be sure to purchase unsweetened, light coconut milk, which is available in most large supermarkets.

COOKING GREENS: These dark, leafy greens are full of beta-carotene, vitamin C, folate, and many other potential cancer-fighting and heart-protecting nutrients. They include beet greens, chard, collards, dandelion greens, kale, mustard greens, spinach, and turnip greens.

QUICK TIP: Look for cooking greens in convenient ready-pack bags. These are washed and torn so all you have to do is sauté them in a little extra virgin olive oil and sprinkle them with salt and pepper. Cooking greens can also be steamed.

SMART COOK: Keep cooking greens and salad greens in your crisper drawer, wrapped in barely dampened paper

towels and placed in a plastic bag; this will help keep them fresh. Use all greens within a few days of purchase.

COOKING SPRAY: See Butter-Flavored Fat-Free Cooking Spray on page 16.

CONDIMENTS: Low-sugar condiments are widely available these days. Try ketchups, teriyaki sauces, jams (Phases 2 and 3 only), and mustards to conveniently enhance dishes made with fresh vegetables, lean proteins, and whole-grain crackers and breads.

COUSCOUS: Tiny grains of semolina make couscous, a central ingredient in North African cuisine and a tasty alternative to rice and other grains. You'll want to purchase whole-wheat couscous, which you can find in health food stores and large supermarkets. Try it in our Chicken Couscous (page 287).

CRACKERS: Whole-grain and multigrain crackers make satisfying snacks. Try them with hummus or a piece of low-fat cheese or use them to make a Green Apple and Peanut Butter Sandwich (page 139).

CUCUMBERS: A crisp, refreshing veggie that is available year-round. You'll find countless uses for cucumbers in our recipes, which include delicious salads and refreshing cold soups. Sliced cucumbers make a great base for spreads such as hummus or a slice of reduced-fat cheese if you're on Phase 1.

CURRY PASTE: This blend of ground curry powder, vinegar, and other spices is often found with Southeast Asian or Thai ingredients in the supermarket; combine it with coconut milk to make tasty soups and fish and chicken stews.

DATES: Fresh or dried, dates are a great source of potassium and fiber and also supply some iron and protein. But remember that they contain a lot of sugar and must be eaten in moderation (three per serving). Dates make a delicious and portable sweet snack, especially when paired with pecans (see Pecan-Stuffed Dates, page 140).

EGGPLANT: This globe-shaped veggie is a favorite Italian ingredient. High in fiber and (like most vegetables) practically fat-free, eggplant is especially good roasted (see Roasted Eggplant with Lemon and Olive Oil, page 430) and baked.

EGGS: A very economical source of protein, eggs are among the fastest cooking foods around! Plus, they are delicious and packed with vitamin B_{12}, riboflavin, and selenium. Most South Beach Diet recipes use large eggs. The yolk does contain many of the nutrients, and recent studies have shown moderate egg consumption to be safe and healthy. However, if you're concerned about your cholesterol, talk to your doctor and monitor your cholesterol while increasing egg consumption.

SMART COOK: Not sure if your eggs are fresh? Fill up a bowl of salted cool water and gently add an egg. If it sinks, it's fresh; if it floats, it's not.

EXTRACTS: These concentrated flavorings are made up of alcohol and extractives that give them flavor, like vanilla or orange. Primarily used in baked goods, extracts are wonderful flavor enhancers; they keep indefinitely when stored in a cool, dry place.

FENNEL: This bulbous, white vegetable is deliciously crisp and adds wonderful flavor to salads as well as fish and meat dishes. When cooked, its bold flavor softens, as you'll see when you try our Pork Chops with Fennel and Lemon (page 360). Look for firm bulbs with straight stalks. You can chop up the fronds and add them to salads and rice dishes as you would a fresh herb.

SMART COOK: Slice (or shave) fennel thinly for eating raw, thicker for sautéing, roasting, or braising. When sliced thinly, the vegetable's flavor is very delicate and tasty; when cooked, it becomes somewhat milder.

FISH AND SHELLFISH: Fish is a great low-fat, lean protein. Since there are so many different types, we don't name them all here—but we give you some of the basic ones that are used in this book and offer substitutes for those times when you find yourself with a limited selection. Because of mercury levels, it's best to limit consumption of canned tuna and swordfish. Fish oil supplements are a safe and healthy way to get the benefits of the omega-3 fatty acids found in fish. Note that high-quality frozen fish is becoming more and more available. It's great when you're looking for ease and convenience, as it makes for easy stocking up.

QUICK TIP: Many frozen fish come seasoned with delightful combinations of herbs and spices; all you have to do is defrost and cook. Avoid breaded versions and remember to thaw frozen fish completely in the refrigerator before using.

• **Anchovies:** These tasty small fish are packed with heart-healthy omega-3 oils. Widely available canned and jarred, they are perfect quick and easy fare. Use them in salads, sandwiches, and pastas.

QUICK TIP: If you're an anchovy enthusiast, look for the puréed paste, sold in a convenient tube for easy long-term use. It's great in pasta sauces, meat marinades, and spreads. A half teaspoon of anchovy paste is equivalent to one anchovy fillet.

• **Catfish:** Named for its whisker-like feelers, this mainly freshwater fish has a firm, white flaky flesh. Low in fat and mild in flavor, catfish can be baked, roasted, pan cooked, steamed, grilled, or cooked in soups or stews. Try Baked Catfish with Lemon Aioli (page 248). You can use snapper or fluke in recipes that call for catfish.

• **Clams:** You can find live clams in the shell, fresh or frozen shucked, or canned (which is a handy convenience product). Live clams should be scrubbed well before cooking to remove the sand that is lodged on their shells. These tasty shellfish are high in protein and offer fair amounts of calcium and iron. For a quick weeknight dinner, try our Spaghetti with White Clam Sauce (page 241).

• **Cod:** This very tasty, lean white fish has a firm texture and a deliciously mild flavor. Try it broiled, baked (see Cod with Artichokes and Basil, page 225) or in Cod Chowder (page 237).

• **Grouper:** A member of the sea bass family, this lean, firm-fleshed fish is found in the Gulf of Mexico and the

North and South Atlantic. It's delicious baked, poached, or steamed. If it's not available, substitute cod, haddock, or striped bass.

• **Mackerel:** A relative of tuna, mackerel is rich in taste and in omega-3s, protein, B vitamins, and the antioxidant selenium. If you've never tried it, our Baked Mackerel Fillets (page 226) is a great place to start. Mackerel is available fresh and canned.

• **Mussels:** Low in fat, high in vitamin B_{12}, and rich in protein, iron, and selenium, mussels are easy to prepare and fun to eat. Try them in our Spicy Mussels with Tomato and Basil (page 231).

• **Salmon:** Protein, thiamin, niacin, omega-3 fatty acids, potassium, and vitamins B_6, B_{12}, and D are just a few of the many health benefits that this beloved fish offers. Salmon is available fresh, smoked, and canned; it's so versatile, you'll find it in breakfast, lunch, and dinner recipes.

• **Sardines:** This underrated fish provides heart-healthy omega-3 fatty acids. Sardines come fresh and canned. Canned versions make fantastic quick dishes, and many even come in their own flavorful tomato or mustard sauces.

• **Shrimp:** This popular shellfish is widely available both fresh and frozen (and already peeled and deveined). Keep the frozen ones on hand so they'll be there when you're ready to defrost and then sauté, grill, steam, or bake them. Shrimp cook up in mere minutes; just don't overcook them or they'll become tough and flavorless.

SMART COOK: If you want to use your frozen shrimp and forgot to defrost them in the refrigerator, place them in a colander and run cool water over them until they thaw.

Note: Shrimp are an exception to the defrosting rule. The safest way to thaw frozen food is in the refrigerator or on the thaw cycle of the microwave. When defrosting frozen foods in the refrigerator, place them on a plate or in an extra plastic bag so they do not leak onto other food items.

• **Trout:** These freshwater fish have a mild, sweet flavor and are wonderful broiled, grilled, or baked. Smoked trout (found in supermarkets near the smoked salmon) makes a tasty addition to tossed green salads or a good snack with crudités and whole-grain crackers.

• **Tuna:** An excellent source of B vitamins, tuna is also rich in omega-3 fatty acids and the mineral selenium. Fresh tuna is as popular as canned. Buy the canned version packed in water.

QUICK TIP: In addition to canned tuna and salmon, many supermarkets now carry vacuum-packed fish in no-drain foil pouches. These mess-free products are tasty and convenient. Perfect for boating or camping or taking to the beach, the office, or school, some brands come with delicious seasonings—you don't even need a can opener!

• **Asian fish sauce (nuoc nam or nam pla):** This common Southeast Asian condiment made of fermented, salted fish adds incomparable flavor to the dishes it's made with. Look for it in the Asian section of your supermarket or health food store, and try it in our tasty

Phase 1 Vietnamese Pork Rolls (page 333), and many other South Beach dishes.

FLOUR: There are more nonwhite flours out there than you probably realize. Once you get to know them, you can incorporate them into your baked and breakfast goods. You can use whole-grain and nonwheat flours in Phases 2 and 3, but avoid all flour in Phase 1.

• **Buckwheat flour:** A great source of fiber, buckwheat is actually not a wheat, but an herb. Milled into a flour, it is used to make soba noodles and is often used in pancake mixes. Buckwheat flour comes in light and dark forms; the dark boasts the most fiber and strongest flavor. You may be familiar with toasty, nutty-flavored kasha, which is roasted, hulled, crushed buckwheat kernels (also known as buckwheat groats). Because it does not contain gluten, buckwheat is a good choice for people allergic to wheat. Try it in our Blueberry Buckwheat Pancakes (page 82).

• **Chickpea flour:** This flavorful flour made from dried, ground chickpeas is nonwheat and gluten-free. You'll find chickpea flour in health food stores, and you can use it in our Savory Egg, Ham, and Cheese Crêpes (page 84).

• **Nut flour:** See Nuts.

• **Whole-wheat flour:** This healthy flour is a great alternative to standard white flour and can be used in place of it in most baked goods.

• **Whole-wheat pastry flour:** This soft whole-wheat flour is better suited for light pastries, muffins, and cakes than denser, regular whole-wheat flour.

Quick and Healthy Fish Cookery

All types of fish and shellfish are recommended on the South Beach Diet. Just avoid breading and frying. Try some of these fast cooking methods for delicious fish.

Sauté. This technique is perfect for all types of fish fillets, including grouper, catfish, haddock, perch, red snapper, tilefish, and weakfish. Simply season the fish, heat 1 tablespoon of extra-virgin olive oil in a skillet over medium-high heat, and cook 2 to 3 minutes per side. Hint: If you love breaded fish, try seasoning fish fillets, then dredging them in toasted, finely crushed nuts before sautéing. Or dredge lightly in whole wheat bread crumbs in Phases 2 or 3.

Poach or steam. To poach, bring water and lemon juice, white wine, or clam juice to a simmer in a large, deep-sided skillet (you want enough liquid to completely cover the fish once added). Add the fish (halibut steaks and grouper, monkfish, and salmon fillets poach especially well; most other fillets will fall apart) and gently simmer until the flesh is opaque, 6 to 12 minutes, depending on the fish. Never boil your cooking liquid when poaching. You can steam fish over a similar liquid for approximately the same amount of time.

Bake. Arrange seasoned fish fillets or steaks in a baking dish, sprinkle with salt and pepper, and drizzle with extra-virgin olive oil. Bake at 400°F for approximately 10 minutes for ¾-inch-thick pieces. Squeeze lemon juice onto the fish before serving or try seasoning with dried herbs or red pepper flakes before cooking. You can also bake shrimp and scallops.

Broil. Season fish, then brush with extra-virgin olive oil, and broil. Good broiling choices include: tuna and other firm steaks, scallops and shrimp, and any type of fillet, including grouper, catfish, haddock, perch, red snapper, tilefish, and weakfish. Cooking times vary. Shrimp and scallops take approximately 2 minutes per side, while fillets generally require 4 or 5 minutes total; steaks require 4 or 5 minutes per side per 1-inch thickness.

Grill. If you love grilled fish but don't want to fuss with an outdoor grill, purchase a cast-iron grill pan. It heats up in minutes, requires little oil, and produces a delicious finished product with those nice grill marks. Fish steaks are best for grilling and generally take 3 to 5 minutes per side. Good choices include grouper, monkfish, salmon, and tuna; shrimp work well, too.

SMART COOK: Because whole-grain and nut flours contain some fat or oil, you'll want to store them in the refrigerator or freezer to prevent them from turning rancid. Keeping flour in the fridge or freezer will also prevent pesky bug infestations.

GARLIC: A beloved medicinal food, garlic is a key ingredient in many savory dishes. Choose solid bulbs, with tight skins.

QUICK TIP: Peeled, minced garlic is a great staple to keep in the fridge—just think of all the time you'll save not having to peel and chop each clove. Note: 1 teaspoon minced garlic is the general equivalent of 1 whole garlic clove.

SMART COOK: If you prefer fresh, whole garlic to the jarred minced version, you'll appreciate this quick and easy peeling technique: Place an unpeeled clove on its side on a cutting board; slice off the end that holds the bulb together. Then place the flat side of a broad knife over the clove and give it a gentle, yet firm whack with the heel of your palm. The peel will split and the clove will easily pop out. Extra hint: Use a garlic press, if you have one, in recipes calling for minced garlic; though it's not a true mince, it makes a great stand-in and is much faster than mincing by hand.

GELATIN: Sugar-free fruit-flavored gelatins make a great sweet treat in all phases. Use them on their own or, in Phases 2 and 3, as a base for fresh fruit gelatin parfaits. We use powdered plain gelatin to make our Chocolate Pudding (page 448).

GRAPEFRUIT: Grapefruit come in pink, white, and red; all provide vitamin C and fiber, and the pink and red contain the antioxidants beta-carotene and lycopene. As with oranges, go for the whole fruit instead of just the juice, since it offers more nutritional benefits and fiber.

GRAPES: Naturally sweet and juicy, grapes make a good snack or dessert. Or try them in our Turkey Salad with Pistachios and Grapes (page 173).

GREEN BEANS (AND YELLOW WAX BEANS): A great source of fiber, green and yellow beans also contain beta-carotene and folate. These beans can be blanched and chopped into salads or drizzled with olive oil and sprinkled with salt and pepper. You can also try roasting, grilling, and stir-frying beans in combination with other vegetables.

QUICK TIP: Trimming beans can be a time-consuming pursuit, but you can often find ready-trimmed beans in the supermarket produce section. Purchase these and you can cross the task right off your prep list.

GUACAMOLE: Although it's easy to prepare at home, you can often purchase fresh, already-made versions of this tasty mash made from avocado, lime juice, onion, and cilantro. Look for it in the refrigerated section of the supermarket.

QUICK TIP: Use store-bought guacamole as a delicious veggie dip for a snack or appetizer and as a tasty, instant sandwich filling.

HALF-AND-HALF: Stick with nonfat half-and-half if you like to lighten your morning coffee (limit yourself to 1 tablespoon per cup). Better yet, try switching to 1 percent milk.

HAM: Boiled ham and turkey ham make great sandwiches and are also delicious chopped into salads. Look for extra-lean ham and remember that any ham cured or processed using honey, brown sugar, or maple syrup is off-limits.

HEARTS OF PALM: True to the name, hearts of palm are the edible inner part of a palm tree's stem. Conveniently canned, they're ready to use. Once opened, store them in their own liquid, in a resealable container in the refrigerator, for up to 1 week. Chop and toss hearts of palm into salads or main dishes.

HERBS: Herbs are a must for cooking full-flavored, delicious dishes. Use dried ones for baked or cooked dishes and the fresh for salads or to garnish finished cooked fish, meats, and pastas. Look for fresh herbs with a vibrant, uniform green color; avoid wilted ones.

- **Basil:** Fresh basil is used whole, torn, or chopped in salads, egg dishes, and pastas. Dried basil is perfect for baked chicken or fish and in soups.

- **Chives:** A relative of onion and leek, chives have a mild onion-like flavor. Snip them with scissors or gently chop with a sharp knife, then try them in chicken salad or scrambled eggs.

- **Cilantro:** This lively tasting herb is popular in Asia, the Caribbean, and Latin America. Use it to make salsas, toss it into salads, or sprinkle it over baked chicken or fish.

- **Mint:** Most people think of mint as an herb used in desserts (like in our Fruit Salad with Lime and Mint, page

459), but it is also terrific in soups and salads. You'll find it used often in this book.

• **Parsley:** Fresh parsley makes a great garnish for cooked meats, chicken, and fish and is tasty in beans, pasta, and rice dishes. You'll find it dried in Italian seasoning and other packaged herb mixes.

• **Rosemary:** There's nothing quite like the piney flavor of this wonderful herb, which is often used to flavor meats, fish, soups, stews, vegetables, sauces, and dressings.

• **Sage:** This Mediterranean herb has a strong earthy flavor that is perfect for chicken, pork, ham, bean, and vegetable dishes.

• **Thyme:** Popular in French dishes, thyme has an assertive flavor that goes well with many foods, including tomato dishes and vegetable soups, as well as meats, poultry, and fish.

QUICK TIP: Enhance your store-bought, low-sugar pasta sauce with a few pinches of dried herbs (thyme, rosemary, and basil are good choices, on their own or in combination), a pinch of freshly ground black pepper or red pepper flakes, and a minced clove of garlic or two. Mix together and gently heat for 10 to 15 minutes before tossing with whole-wheat pasta or using in baked dishes.

QUICK TIP: Don't let leftover fresh herbs wither away in the back of the produce drawer! Instead use them to make your own dried herbs by placing them in a single layer on a baking pan; place the pan in the oven with just the light on (no heat) for 12 to 24 hours (put a note on the oven door so

you remember to remove them before using the oven). Then simply crush and store them in small glass jars. You'll be amazed at how flavorful your freshly dried herbs are—and it just takes a few active minutes of your time.

SMART COOK: Dried herbs (store-bought or home-dried), like spices, should be kept in a cool, dry place and used within 6 months of purchase. After this time, they will rapidly begin to lose flavor and pungency.

SMART COOK: To store fresh herbs, wrap them in barely dampened paper towels, place them in a resealable plastic bag that is just partially sealed, and refrigerate for 3 to 7 days. Some varieties, like parsley and rosemary, keep longer than others, like basil.

SMART COOK: Try growing a small pot of one or two fresh herbs on your windowsill; as long as you keep them trimmed and well watered, the delicious fresh leaves will be there for you anytime!

HORSERADISH: Enhance sauces, spreads, salad dressings, and even sandwiches with convenient prepared horseradish. It comes jarred in the refrigerated section of the supermarket. You can also purchase this spicy herb fresh in the produce section and grate it yourself. Look for firm, unblemished roots. We use it to make a zippy cream for steak in our Peppery Steak with Horseradish Cream (page 355); the cream is great on fish, too.

HOT DOGS: Hot dogs (beef, pork, poultry, and soy) can make very quick and easy meals (Phases 2 and 3 only). Just stick to products that are 97 percent fat-free

(3 to 6 grams of fat per serving) and enjoy them occasionally, no more than once a week. Go for whole-grain buns or eat them without a bun, with sauerkraut, sugar-free pickle relish, and Dijon mustard.

HUMMUS: This thick Middle Eastern purée of chickpeas, garlic, fresh lemon juice, and olive oil makes a fantastic quick snack (with crudités or whole-grain crackers) and sandwich filling. Look for hummus canned or fresh in your supermarket's refrigerated section or deli.

QUICK TIP: Keep hummus, sliced pepper strips, and celery sticks in the fridge at your office for a satisfying, no-cook midday snack.

JAM: There are many delicious low-sugar jams on the market these days. Use them in Phases 2 and 3.

KALE: This cruciferous cooking green is rich in fiber, vitamin C, vitamin B$_6$, and beta-carotene; it also provides calcium. Sauté kale with garlic and extra-virgin olive oil. And also try Turkey Sausages with Kale and Chickpeas (page 272) and Lentil and Kale Stew (page 403).

KASHA: A toasty, nutty-flavored grain, kasha is buckwheat kernels that have been roasted and hulled. Because it does not contain gluten, kasha is a good choice for people allergic to wheat. Look for kasha in the cereal (not the grain) aisle in supermarkets and health food stores; it is often eaten for breakfast but equally enjoyed as an ingredient in grain and side dishes. We even use it in a filling for our Veggie Burrito (page 380).

KEBABS: In a good supermarket, the butcher will offer lean cuts of chicken, beef, and pork already cut into kebab pieces for you. This will help you save prep time at home. You might also find marinated kebabs (and other cuts of meat), which are very convenient—just make sure they are sugar-free.

QUICK TIP: Purchase low-sugar marinades for meats, vegetables, tempeh, and tofu or quickly make your own at home using fresh garlic, dried herbs, extra-virgin olive oil, and a little balsamic vinegar. For an Asian marinade, combine soy sauce, sesame oil, freshly grated or ground ginger, and minced garlic.

LAMB: Although flavorful, lamb is a fattier meat than many others. Be sure to buy a well-trimmed boneless leg.

LEMONS: An excellent source of vitamin C, this citrus fruit is a delicious flavor enhancer for dressings, marinades, savory dishes, and desserts.

LIMES: Another popular citrus fruit and also filled with vitamin C, a lime lends terrific flavor to all kinds of dishes.

QUICK TIP: Skip the work of squeezing fresh lemons and limes every time you need them by preparing both juices in advance. Use an electric or hand juicer (or your hands) to juice a dozen of each fruit and then pour the juice into ice cube trays. Once frozen, transfer the juice cubes to freezer bags and store in the freezer. When needed, simply remove one or two cubes and thaw in the microwave for your instant "freshly squeezed" juice! Remember that fruit at room temperature will yield more juice than fruit that is cold.

QUICK TIP: Lemon or lime zest—the colored, flavorful peel—can enhance the flavor of many dishes. Invest in a zesting tool to remove zest fastest. Make sure you scrub the fruit thoroughly before removing the zest and avoid the bitter white pith underneath.

MANGOES: This aromatic tropical fruit is juicy and flavorful. An excel-lent source of beta-carotene, mangoes also provide soluble fiber and vitamin C.

MAYONNAISE: Used sparingly, mayonnaise makes delicious sandwich spreads and salads. Use mayonnaise on its own or to make a quick aioli—a French condiment that combines mayonnaise with minced garlic. See Baked Catfish with Lemon Aioli (page 248). Purchase mayonaise regular, reduced-fat, or dairy-free (soy-based, without eggs). Avoid fat-free varieties or those made with high-fructose corn syrup.

MELONS: A wonderful source of potassium, vitamin C, and B vitamins, melons are mildly sweet. They make a delicious breakfast or dessert fruit, as in Fruit Salad with Lime and Mint (page 459) and Melon Slush (page 479).

MESCLUN: Also marketed as spring mix, mesclun is a mixture of baby salad greens that often includes arugula, dandelion, frisée, oak leaf, and radicchio.

MILK: Milk is an important source of protein, calcium, and vitamins A, D, and B_{12}. Choose fat-free or 1 percent milk, which contain the same nutrients as whole milk, without as much fat.

MIRIN: This low-alcohol cooking wine made from glutinous rice adds a sweet flavor to Japanese dishes. Mirin, also referred to as rice wine, can be found in the Asian section of most supermarkets and in health food stores and Japanese markets. You can make a substitute for mirin by adding 2 tablespoons of granular sugar substitute to 1 cup of dry white wine. Stir mixture together well and keep refrigerated for up to 1 month.

MISO PASTE: Made from fermented soybeans, this flavorful, protein-rich Japanese staple can be found in the Asian section of most health food stores and many supermarkets. Use it to make quick soups, like Hearty Miso Soup with Soba (page 389), or as a marinade for fish, poultry, or meat.

MUSTARD: We use mustards liberally on South Beach because they're such terrific and convenient flavor enhancers for meats and fish. Try regular Dijon and coarse-grain Dijon in many of the recipes in this book, including Mustard-Crusted Steak (page 327). Avoid honey mustards or any others that contain sugar.

MUSHROOMS: A good source of dietary fiber, mushrooms also provide niacin, riboflavin, iron, potassium, and selenium. Delicious raw and cooked, mushrooms are terrific in salads as well as in sautéed and baked dishes.

NUTS: High in protein and very satisfying, dry-roasted nuts make a great snack and add a wonderful crunch to salads and rice dishes. They also show up in extracts, desserts, and sauces and are used to make oils, butters, and flour. Nut flour contains no actual flour at all; it's simply the solids of previously pressed nuts ground into a flour-like powder. And nut butters? They go far beyond peanut butter. Look for almond, cashew, and peanut butters that are both sugar- and trans fat-free. Remember to stick to recommended portion sizes, as nuts are high in calories.

QUICK TIP: For extra flavor, toast nuts in a skillet, stirring often, over a very low flame or in a 325°F oven for 5 to 10 minutes. Add toasted nuts to salads or sprinkle them over pasta and fish dishes.

SMART COOK: Store nuts in a closed plastic container in the refrigerator or freezer, where they are safe from becoming rancid.

• **Almonds:** Rich in vitamin E, these heart-healthy nuts also offer protein, riboflavin, iron, and magnesium and are higher in fiber than most other nuts.

QUICK TIP: Coarsely grind a handful of almonds, hazelnuts, pistachios, or pine nuts in a food processor, mix with your favorite dried herbs, and use it to coat any kind of fish fillet. Then season with salt and pepper and bake until golden.

• **Cashews:** Lower in total fat than most nuts and seeds, cashews deliver big when it comes to iron, vitamin E, magnesium, and zinc (and also to taste!). Still, they are relatively high in saturated fat, so (as always) stick to portion sizes.

• **Hazelnuts:** Wonderful sweet nuts, popular in both savory dishes and desserts, hazelnuts have monounsaturated fats that are presumed to be helpful in lowering LDL ("bad") cholesterol levels. They also have contain of the nutrients associated with other nuts.

- **Macadamia nuts:** Widely grown in Hawaii, these pale, round nuts have a slightly sweet, creamy flavor. Since they contain both a high fat and calorie content, stick to eight per serving.

- **Peanuts:** Though used and thought of as nuts, peanuts are actually legumes. Their nutritional benefits include very high protein, vitamin E, folate, niacin, and magnesium. Just a small amount of chopped peanuts delivers a big flavor to dishes like Peanut Chicken with Noodles (page 285).

- **Peanut butter:** High in monounsaturated fat, folate, and resveratrol (the phytochemical found in red wine that helps protect against heart disease and cancer), peanut butter is wonderful in desserts like Peanut Butter and Jelly Cookies (page 453). You can enjoy it spread onto celery for a healthy, portable, hunger-curbing snack—even in Phase 1. Limit peanut butter to 2 tablespoons per serving; purchase natural and sugar-free varieties only.

- **Pecans:** Heart-healthy fat abounds in pecans, which also offer thiamin, zinc, and fiber.

- **Pine nuts:** Also known as pignoli or piñon nuts, pine nuts are the seeds of pinecones. Delicious in salads, pastas, and baked goods, they keep best in an airtight container in the refrigerator for up to 3 months, or frozen for up to 9 months.

- **Pistachios:** Another heart-healthy nut, pistachios offer cholesterol-lowering fats, plus nutritional benefits that include fiber, vitamin E, iron, thiamin, and magnesium. Sprinkle them over salads, chicken dishes, and desserts.

• **Walnuts:** Walnuts are unique in the nut world in that they contain a heart-healthy omega-3 acid called alpha-linolenic acid, as well as many other nutritional benefits. You'll find them in our salads (see Green Leaf, Pear, and Goat Cheese Salad, page 181) as well as in breakfast dishes and desserts.

OATS: This flavor-packed grain is incredibly nutritious, offering 50 percent more protein than bulgur wheat and twice as much as brown rice. But that's not all: Oats have an impressively high soluble-fiber content (good for lowering LDL cholesterol) and provide thiamin, iron, selenium, magnesium, and zinc. Choose steel-cut oats over instant-cook oatmeal (which is too highly processed). You'll enjoy them in our Spiced Oatmeal with Dried Apricot and Walnuts (page 88).

QUICK TIP: Prepare oatmeal ahead of time and refrigerate for up to 5 days. When it's time for breakfast, simply microwave for about 3 minutes with 1 percent or skim milk or low-fat, low-sugar plain or vanilla soymilk and enjoy!

OILS: Oils are extremely important ingredients, especially in South Beach recipes, where you'll use them to cook, make simple dressings, and drizzle over mouthwatering meats, fish, and vegetables. You'll want to store most oils in a cool, dark pantry (except for nut oils, which belong in the fridge).

• **Canola oil:** Lower in saturated fat than any other oil, canola oil offers the benefit of omega-3 fatty acids, which are helpful in both brain development and the reduction of cholesterol. Canola oil is perfect for cooking and for salad dressings.

- **Extra-virgin olive oil:** The most flavorful and fruity of the olive oils, extra-virgin olive oil can be used for cooking and for salad dressings.

- **Flavored oils:** You'll find herb and other flavored olive oils in your market. These can enhance your simple salad dressings or even a plate of your favorite grilled or roasted vegetables.

- **Nut oils:** These delicate oils are delicious for use in salads or drizzled over cooked vegetables (they're not meant for cooking). They come both roasted and unroasted. Look for roasted nut oils (which are stronger in flavor than the unroasted) in specialty and gourmet stores, where you'll find almond oil, hazelnut oil, pecan oil, and walnut oil, among many others. Once opened, nut oils must be kept in the refrigerator or they will quickly turn rancid.

- **Sesame oil:** This delicious full-flavored Asian oil is made from sesame seeds; it's used often in South Beach recipes, like Sesame Green Beans, page 416, and many others. Look for dark or regular sesame oil in the Asian section at most supermarkets, and store it in a cool, dry place.

OLIVES: These small, flavor-packed fruits make a fantastic snack, appetizer, and salad ingredient; they also taste great in pastas as well as meat and fish dishes. Olives contain healthy monounsaturated fatty acids, which may help to lower "bad" LDL cholesterol. When using olives, remember to stick to recommended portion sizes.

QUICK TIP: Look for marinated olives, which are often flavored with dried herbs, fresh garlic, citrus peel, or red pepper flakes. Eat them as snacks or use them to flavor pastas, salads, and meat, poultry, fish, and even rice dishes. They'll do the work of adding extra flavor to your meals, and you won't have to get out the herbs and spices. You can also look for jarred olive salad, which generally consists of pitted, chopped olives flavored with olive oil and salad vegetables.

ONIONS: Keep onions (including red, white, Spanish or yellow, and scallions) on hand; you'll find them in many South Beach recipes because they are great flavor enhancers. Store whole onions in a cool, dry pantry space, away from bright light and potatoes (which will cause spoilage). Keep scallions in a sealed plastic bag in the refrigerator.

ORANGES: Good sources of vitamin C, folate, and fiber, oranges make a good portable snack and a nice salad ingredient. As with grapefruit, go for the whole fruit in lieu of just the juice; you'll get better nutritional benefits.

PAPAYAS: These somewhat exotic tropical fruits offer vitamins C and E, fiber, folate, potassium, and beta-carotene. Look for all-yellow, yellow-orange, or yellow and green speckled specimens (completely green papayas are not ripe); the flesh of a ripe papaya will give slightly (like an avocado) when gently pressed.

PASTA: Use whole-wheat or spelt pastas, which are flavorful, nutrient rich, and readily available in health food stores or the health food section of large supermarkets.

QUICK TIP: To quickly boil water for pasta, cover your saucepan with a lid; then remove the lid and cook the pasta.

QUICK TIP: Instead of cooking pasta and your fresh or frozen vegetables separately, add the veggies to the pasta cooking water during the last few minutes of cooking. Both will be ready at the same time.

PEANUT BUTTER: See Nuts on page 38.

PEAS: Available fresh and frozen, peas are sweet and tasty. Reintroduce them in Phase 2.

QUICK TIP: Frozen peas are a quick cook's favorite. They are very high in quality and (depending on the dish) do not even require thawing. Toss them with hot whole-wheat pasta, olive oil, fresh lemon juice, and salt and pepper, for example.

QUICK TIP: Frozen produce is a quick and easy alternative to fresh. Don't worry about missing out on nutrients; generally vegetables and fruits are frozen upon harvest, when their nutrient levels are highest. You can store frozen fruits and vegetables up to 8 or even 12 months—simply pull them out when you're ready to use them.

PEARS: A good source of fiber, pears are higher in sugar than many other fruits. Enjoy them in moderation or in combination with other foods.

PEPPERS: Sweet peppers offer vitamins B_6 and C and also provide fiber; hot ones are a good source of vitamin

C. Both add delicious flavor to many dishes; raw sweet peppers also make a good snack and salad ingredient. Jarred, roasted red peppers are widely available and are a key ingredient when it comes to convenience and in quick-cook dishes.

PICKLES: Pickles make a tangy and delicious easy side dish at barbecues and picnics. If you are watching your sodium, use only very moderate amounts. No-sugar-added pickles and pickle relishes are available in many supermarkets.

PESTO: This blend of fresh basil, pine nuts, Parmesan cheese, and olive oil is delicious and can be tossed with pasta or drizzled over meats and fish to create quick, no-fuss meals. You can even mix it into lean ground pork to make a delicious burger (see Stuffed Pork Burger, page 362) or combine it with reduced-fat sour cream for a tasty dip. Convenient store-bought pesto is widely available.

PHYLLO: The Greek word for "leaf," phyllo is a tissue-thin dough used in Greek dishes such as spanakopita as well as desserts (including our Thin and Crispy Pear Tart, page 450). You'll find whole-wheat phyllo (avoid the white version) in the freezer section of supermarkets and health food stores. Enjoy it in Phases 2 and 3.

POMEGRANATE: This beautiful fruit bears delicious seeds and also offers an impressive and concentrated source of antioxidant phytochemicals. Pomegranates also provide vitamins B_6 and C as well as potassium. Use the seeds in salads and rice, poultry, and pork dishes. When choosing pomegranates, look for specimens with shiny, unbroken skins; store them in the refrigerator for up to 2 months.

SMART COOK: To seed a pomegranate, cut off the crown end, then score the rind in quarters from top to bottom. Place the fruit in a large bowl of cool water, gently pull the sections apart, and remove the seeds with your fingers; discard the thin membrane and the outer skin. Drain and refrigerate the seeds in an airtight container for up to 3 days. The whole seed of a pomegranate is edible.

PORK: Lean cuts of pork (chops, cutlets, loin, and tenderloin) are wonderful, tasty forms of protein. Though you should stay away from regular bacon and hams cured with honey, you can eat moderate amounts of Canadian bacon and boiled ham; you can also have turkey and soy bacons.

POULTRY: Choose skinless chicken breasts or chicken cutlets, which are high in protein and low in fat. Already-cooked (usually poached or grilled) strips, skinless breasts, and cutlets can be found in the refrigerated section and the deli case at well-stocked supermarkets, reducing your prep time on many recipes—they can practically go straight from the package to your plate! Look for grilled chicken strips and oven-roasted chicken cuts. Turkey bacon and reduced-fat turkey sausages are fine, but avoid duck and goose, as well as dark meat chicken and turkey (legs and wings), since these are high in fat. Also avoid processed poultry nuggets and patties.

QUICK TIP: When you're doing the shopping for a stuffed beef, pork, or poultry recipe, ask your butcher to cut pockets into chops or chicken breasts for you. This free service will save you valuable time in the kitchen.

QUINOA: Pronounced "keen-wah," this small, sand-colored, grain-like product (a relative of leafy vegetables like spinach) contains all nine essential amino acids necessary for the body to function, as well as more protein and fewer carbohydrates than any grain. It is grown in South America, has a deliciously mild flavor, and can be substituted for rice or grains in many recipes. Try our Quinoa Pilaf (page 418).

RADISHES: These crisp and crunchy root vegetables are high in potassium and vitamin C. Try them sliced into salads or on their own as a snack or appetizer.

RASPBERRIES: A good source of fiber and vitamin C, raspberries also contain antioxidants. They make a great breakfast, snack, salad, or dessert ingredient. Raspberries are available fresh or frozen (avoid frozen versions that contain added sugar); you can also freeze your own.

QUICK TIP: Freeze fresh berries in a single layer on a baking sheet or in a baking dish; once frozen, transfer to a resealable freezer bag, label, date, and store in the freezer until ready to use.

RICE: See Brown Rice on page 14.

RICE VINEGAR: See Vinegars on page 56.

RICE WINE: See Mirin on page 38.

ROAST BEEF: As long as you choose fat-free or low-fat roast beef, you can use this handy deli meat in sandwiches or snacks.

ROASTED RED PEPPERS: See Peppers on page 44.

SALAD DRESSING: In this book, we offer many easy, heart-healthy salad dressings using extra-virgin olive oil and vinegar or fresh lemon juice. They are featured with the salad recipes (not in a dressing and condiment section). Use any of these dressings for your favorite salads or purchase low-sugar varieties that contain no more than 3 grams of sugar per serving. Remember to steer clear of low-fat salad dressings, which are often high in sugars and unhealthy processed ingredients.

SALAD GREENS: There are so many delicious varieties of salad greens available, and many of them come washed, torn into bite-size pieces, packaged, and ready to go. Look for spring mix (or mesclun greens), spinach, baby spinach, and romaine.

SALSA: This popular mix of chopped tomatoes, onions, chiles, and cilantro comes conveniently canned, jarred, and fresh (in the refrigerated section of many supermarkets). A fantastic snack with crudités or baked whole-wheat tortillas, salsa also makes a surprising addition to both our Mexican Chicken Soup (page 120) and our Shrimp Gazpacho (page 132). Both recipes illustrate ways to successfully use salsa in place of fresh-cut vegetables.

SALT: Salt comes from either salt mines or the sea. Using a small amount of salt in cooking helps to enhance flavors and reduce bitterness and acidity. Table salt is the most basic type used for cooking, though some prefer kosher, coarse, or specialty salts. Salt can be stored indefinitely in the cupboard.

SAUSAGES: Sausages make quick meals on their own or sliced into pastas. Look for lean turkey (the leanest) or chicken sausages. You'll want to read labels carefully and avoid fillers, like sugars, fats, and bread crumbs. Wellshire Farms (www.wellshirefarms.com) makes great lower-fat sausages that are a good bet.

STRAWBERRIES: High in vitamin C and fiber, these sweet beloved berries make a great breakfast or snack and are delicious in desserts (like our Creamy Dreamy Strawberry Vanilla Shake, page 466). Buy them fresh in season or frozen year-round.

SOBA NOODLES: These Japanese noodles are made of buckwheat and wheat flours (see Buckwheat on page 15 for nutritional information). Eat them hot or cold, combined with chicken, vegetables, or tofu and soy sauce or sesame oil. Look for soba noodles in the Asian section of most well-stocked grocery and health food stores.

SOYMILK: A great source of protein, soymilk also contains B vitamins and iron. Use low-fat, low-sugar soymilk on low-sugar cereals and in smoothies; try it in our Soy Chai Tea, Two Ways (page 142). Convenient boxed packages store well in the pantry so you can always have some on hand. Make sure to purchase low-fat plain soymilk (with 4 grams of fat or less per 8-ounce serving; be sure the product does not contain high-fructose corn syrup).

SOY SAUCE: Made with fermented soybeans, wheat, water, and salt, soy sauce can be used to flavor poultry, fish, and meat, as well as vegetables, sauces, soups, and marinades. Purchase the low-sodium version only.

SPELT: An ancient cereal grain, spelt is high in fiber, protein, and B vitamins. It's easily digestible and often well tolerated by people with wheat allergies. Try nutty spelt pasta, which is available in health food stores and the health food section of some supermarkets.

SPICES: These aromatic seasonings come from the bark, buds, fruit, roots, seeds, or stems of plants and trees. Generally, all spices that don't contain added sugar are recommended on the South Beach Diet. Using them in your cooking is an easy—and quick—way to add more flavor to food. Buy spices ground or whole and store them in a cool, dark place for up to 6 months. The ones listed below are used in this book and are generally quite good to have on hand. Feel free to add your own favorites if you don't see them listed here.

• **Allspice:** A warm, sweet spice, allspice tastes like a mix of cinnamon, nutmeg, and clove. It can be purchased whole or ground and used in both savory and sweet dishes.

• **Cayenne:** This spicy seasoning, made from ground dried cayenne chile peppers, works well in meat and fish dishes, as well as chili and spicy soups.

• **Chili powder:** Chili powder generally refers to a blend that often contains ground chile peppers, cumin, garlic powder, and salt. You'll also find pure chili powders (like Ancho chile pepper), which will be labeled as such.

• **Cinnamon:** This bittersweet spice is wonderful in baked goods and also makes appearances in savory dishes (especially in Greek and Moroccan cuisines). Sprinkle it onto sweet potatoes and winter squash before baking.

• **Cumin:** Very common in Mexican, Indian, and Tex-Mex cooking, cumin is a heady spice with an aromatic scent. It is delicious in both meat and vegetable dishes.

• **Garam masala:** It makes sense that garam masala means "blend" in the Indian language, as it is a wonderful mixture of ground coriander, black pepper, cardamom, cinnamon, cloves, ginger, and nutmeg. It may also include other spices, such as fennel. You can blend your own version, of course, but it's most convenient to buy it already blended.

• **Garlic powder:** This fine powder adds strong garlic flavor to sauces and meat dishes.

• **Ginger:** Wonderful in desserts as well as savory dishes, this warming, piquant spice is available fresh and ground.

QUICK TIP: Use a spoon to quickly scrape the papery skin off fresh ginger (if the skin is thin, you don't need to peel it) and quickly grate it with a Microplane or box grater. Tightly wrap whole pieces of fresh ginger in plastic and store it in the produce drawer for up to 3 weeks or in the freezer (in a freezer bag) for up to a year.

- **Nutmeg:** Another sweet spice, nutmeg is sold whole and ground.

- **Pepper:** This popular spice comes whole and ground in black, white, green, and pink varieties. Grind whole peppercorns as you need them for the freshest taste.

- **Paprika:** A dried version of mild to hot Spanish peppers, this spice is known for lending flavor and color to savory dishes. You'll find sweet, bittersweet, hot, and smoked paprika, all of which are delicious.

- **Red pepper flakes:** Great for sprinkling onto pasta and other Italian dishes, red pepper flakes are also used to spice up savory Asian dishes.

QUICK TIP: Seasoning blends offer a convenient all-in-one way to flavor meats and fish. From Creole, taco, barbecue, and seafood to mesquite, lemon-pepper blends, and more, these seasonings can be sprinkled onto meats and fish before cooking, shaken onto air-popped popcorn, or mixed with reduced-fat sour cream or yogurt to make quick dips. Remember to check the labels and avoid any that contain sugar or corn syrup.

SPAGHETTI SAUCE: Convenient low-sugar spaghetti sauces come in many flavors. Or get plain sauce and flavor it with fresh garlic and your favorite herbs and spices.

SPELT: See Pasta on page 44.

SPRING MIX: See Mesclun on page 37.

STIR-FRY MIX: See Broccoli on page 14.

SUGAR-FREE PANCAKE SYRUP: Suitable for buckwheat or whole-grain pancakes (which you can enjoy in

Phase 3), this syrup will also give extra flavor to our tasty Phase 1 morning dish Breakfast Turkey Stack (page 78).

SUGAR: Try to avoid white sugar when following the South Beach Diet. However, a small amount of regular sugar may be introduced in Phase 3 as an ingredient in baked goods, for an occasional treat. Remember to monitor yourself for the return of cravings if you do eat sugar.

SUGAR SUBSTITUTE: Use any of the following no-calorie sweeteners: aspartame (Equal), sucralose (Splenda), saccharin (Sprinkle Sweet, Sweet'n Low, Sweet-10), or ace-sulfame K (Sweet One). Stevia is not recommended, as it is not FDA-approved.

SUN-DRIED TOMATOES: Usually packed in oil, these tangy treats enhance sauces, soups, and salads. Buy a low-sodium version, if you can find it.

TAHINI: This thick, rich paste made from sesame seeds is most commonly used to flavor Middle Eastern dishes, like hummus and baba ghanoush. After opening, store tahini in a tightly sealed jar in the refrigerator for up to 3 months.

TAMARI: A wheat-free soy sauce made by aging soybeans, sea salt, and water in wooden casks, tamari has a richer taste than regular soy sauce. Use it to flavor vegetarian dishes, soups, salads, and dressings.

TAPENADE: A thick paste usually made from olives, olive oil, lemon juice, capers, anchovies, and seasonings, tapenade can be used as a topping for fish and poultry, tossed into whole-wheat pasta dishes, brushed onto grilled vegetables, or spread onto sandwiches.

TEA: Tea is not just a morning drink; it also makes a wonderful drink later in the day—try our Soy Chai Tea, Two Ways (page 142). Tea can even be an ingredient in desserts, as in Green Tea Truffles (page 442). Limit caffeinated teas to two cups per day.

TEMPEH: A high-protein mixture of fermented soybeans formed into a cake with a smoky or nutty flavor, tempeh is a great source of vitamin B_{12}. Frozen tempeh keeps well for several months; thawed, it will keep in the refrigerator for about 10 days. Since it's fermented like cheese, tempeh may develop some harmless mold on the surface. Simply cut it away, just as you would on cheese.

TEXTURED VEGETABLE PROTEIN (TVP): This defatted soy flour is a nutrient-rich vegetarian substitute for ground meat. It absorbs flavors well and lends a full-bodied texture to vegetarian burgers, spaghetti sauces, and chili. TVP is a brand name for textured soy protein (TSP), so you can purchase them interchangeably. Look for TVP at health food stores.

TOFU: Made from soymilk curd, which is pressed into small blocks (similar to the way that cheese is made), tofu is rich in iron and is also a good source of protein. Tofu comes in silken and regular varieties, which in turn are divided into soft, firm, and extra firm. Silken tofu is smoother and generally better for baking or smoothies; regular is more granular in texture. The type you use will depend on what you plan to cook. It's a good idea to have firm and extra firm handy for stir-fries and omelets.

TOMATILLOS: Also known as Mexican tomatoes, tomatillos look like small green tomatoes with papery husks. Tangy and slightly lemony and herbaceous, their pronounced flavor softens when cooked. Look for firm specimens, with tight-fitting husks. When ready to cook, simply remove the papery covering with your fingers; the naturally sticky coating underneath will wash off with water.

TOMATOES: Widely used and very popular, tomatoes provide fiber, B vitamins, iron, potassium, and vitamin C. Tomatoes also provide lycopene, a vitamin-like substance that has been shown to help reduce the risk of prostate cancer, cardiovascular disease, and other cancers. They are available fresh, canned, and in sun-dried form (see Sun-Dried Tomatoes on page 53). Canned varieties include Italian and Mexican diced, stewed, diced, whole, and crushed.

TORTILLAS: Whole-wheat tortillas offer a great way to make wraps, quesadillas (see South Beach Eggsadilla, page 93), and even baked chips (see Creamy Tex-Mex Bean Dip with Baked Tortilla Chips, page 150). You can also try sprouted-grain tortillas, which—made from sesame seeds, soybeans, sprouted barley, millet, lentils, and spelt—are 100 percent flourless (try Ezekiel brand, available at health food markets and at www.foodforlife.com).

TRANS-FAT-FREE MARGARINE (OR LIGHT AND REDUCED-FAT SPREADS): While made with vegetable oil and a better choice than butter, trans-fat-free margarine still contains polyunsaturated fat, so use it in moderation. Spreads made with canola oil contain heart-healthy omega-3 oils. Avoid those that contain hydrogenated oils.

TURKEY: Roasted turkey breast, plain or smoked, is available in most delis. You can ask for extra-thick slices and then cube them at home to make salads like Turkey Salad with Pistachios and Grapes (page 173). Turkey hot dogs and turkey bacon are also great quick meal staples.

VINEGARS: Vinegars add a bright, jazzy flavor to marinades and quick dressings. These are just a few of the most popular varieties.

- **Balsamic vinegar:** This flavorful, slightly sweet Italian vinegar is aged in wooden barrels. Mix it with olive oil, herbs, and garlic to make a great marinade for meats.

- **Champagne vinegar:** As its name implies, this soft-tasting wine vinegar is made from Champagne.

- **Cider vinegar:** Made from the fermented juice of pressed apples, this pungent, acidic vinegar is lovely on steamed vegetables and in fresh salads.

- **Flavored vinegars:** You'll find herb- and garlic-flavored vinegars in larger supermarkets and gourmet stores.

- **Rice vinegar:** Made from fermented rice, this mild, slightly sweet vinegar is often used in Japanese and Chinese cooking. We use it in our Tempeh Stir-Fry (page 401) and many other recipes. Look for rice vinegar in the Asian section at health food stores and most large supermarkets.

- **Wine vinegars:** These basic, sharp-tasting vinegars come in red and white.

WORCESTERSHIRE SAUCE: Though first bottled in Worcester, England, this thin, dark sauce has flavor tones reminiscent of India, where it was developed. It is usually made of anchovies, vinegar, molasses, lime, onions, soy sauce, tamarind, and garlic or cloves and is used to season meat, soups, and other dishes. Use it to make your own South Beach Barbecue Sauce (page 309).

YOGURT: High in calcium, yogurt also provides protein, B vitamins, and minerals. This versatile ingredient is great for breakfast, as a snack or dessert, and in sauces. In Phase 1, enjoy plain fat-free or low-fat yogurt. In later phases, you can incorporate artificially sweetened, fat-free flavored yogurts as long as you avoid products that contain high-fructose corn syrup.

ZUCCHINI: A good source of vitamin C, fiber, potassium, and magnesium, this green summer squash makes a tasty addition to many savory South Beach dishes.

Quick Meals You Can Make without a Recipe

Having a bevy of ideas for meals you can make without the constraints of a recipe keeps things extra simple and is a quick way to use up stray ingredients in your refrigerator. That's why I've included the following South Beach snacks and meals that you can easily put together in next to no time. Many of these ideas will help you get a meal together in just 5 or 10 minutes; others might take longer from start to finish, but the time is largely inactive.

Use these ideas as written or just as a springboard for your own recipes, mixing and matching various South Beach-friendly ingredients spontaneously. Learning to improvise with healthy ingredients will make maintaining a South Beach lifestyle even easier!

• Spread Dijon mustard and a touch of mayonnaise on your favorite lean cold cuts and wrap them around crisp lettuce, sliced tomato, and a slice of reduced-fat cheese for a quick, bread-free sandwich or snack.

• A cooked lean hot dog (tucked into a whole-grain bun in Phases 2 and 3 only) with mustard and sauerkraut makes a quick and yummy major-league dinner when served with a salad (try Eggless Caesar Salad, page 161).

• Make an open-faced quesadilla: Place a whole-wheat tortilla on a baking sheet; top with rinsed and drained canned black or pinto beans, 1 ounce of reduced-fat shredded cheese, and fresh or jarred salsa. Bake at 325°F for 5 or 10 minutes.

• Think beyond Tex-Mex! You can make mini pizzas by spreading a thin layer of pesto or low-sugar pasta sauce on a whole-wheat tortilla. Then add thinly sliced skim-milk mozzarella or reduced-fat cheddar cheese and frozen spinach or broccoli florets; bake at 400°F until hot and bubbly.

• Use whole-wheat tortillas to make quick wraps, mixing and matching ingredients like sliced sun-dried tomatoes, a tablespoon or two of olive salad, a drizzle of pesto, or a dollop of prepared guacamole or hummus with veggies or lean cold cuts.

• Use convenient pouch-packed tuna and salmon to make quick salads and sandwiches at the office or on a picnic (or while boating or fishing!). You can purchase already-flavored fish and eat it on its own or with whole-grain crackers and veggie sticks. Or toss the fish with mayonnaise and a blended seasoning (like Cajun) or jarred olive salad or chopped sun-dried tomatoes. No draining necessary.

• Mix together cooked chicken strips and convenient ready-pack salad greens to make a tasty chicken and greens salad. Just toss with 3 parts of extra-virgin olive oil to 1 part of your favorite vinegar or fresh lemon juice; you can even add a pinch or two of blended seasoning and some shredded reduced-fat cheese.

• Grill just about any type of fresh fish steak, drizzle with olive oil, and serve with salad or a favorite vegetable. You can stock your freezer with many kinds of the high-quality frozen fish that are available in supermarkets so you don't have to make a last-minute trip to the market when you want fish for dinner.

• Top any type of fish fillet with fresh salsa, drizzle with extra-virgin olive oil, season with salt and pepper, and bake until opaque throughout.

• Make a cold meal out of packaged salad greens tossed with fresh lemon juice and extra-virgin olive oil, alongside store-bought tabbouli, hummus, and baba ghanoush. Dip vegetable sticks into the two spreads.

• Toss diced chicken strips with mayonnaise, chopped celery, cilantro, and a few sprinklings of packaged dry taco seasoning.

• Toss smoked trout with ready-pack salad greens, fresh lemon juice, and olive oil for a quick high-protein salad. Or mix it with lightly beaten eggs for a tasty smoked trout scramble. Smoked trout is rich in both protein and flavor, making for very satisfying meals.

• Smoked salmon comes thinly sliced and ready to use in convenient small packages. Eat it on top of whole-grain toast spread with reduced-fat cream cheese for breakfast, snacks, or lunch. Or bring reduced-fat cream cheese to room temperature, mix with dried dill and freshly ground black pepper, and spread on a piece of salmon; roll up and eat. This makes a tasty quick snack or appetizer; you can also place two or three alongside a simple salad. Other quick ideas using smoked salmon: Use it in wraps or cut it into pieces and toss into pastas or egg scrambles.

• Eggs make great quick lunch or dinner fare, especially in hot weather when you don't want to crank up the stove. Try them poached over spinach salad tossed with crispy turkey bacon. Or make an omelet with thinly sliced cooked chicken strips, chopped tomato, and ready-pack shredded cheese.

• The high-quality, lower-sodium broths that have become so widely available are perfect for quick homemade soups. Heat some extra-virgin olive oil in a saucepan and add chopped onion, minced garlic, and chopped celery; cook until softened. Add broth, bring to a simmer, and add thinly sliced cooked chicken strips and a few frozen veggies or some cooked rice. Heat until all the ingredients are hot and then enjoy.

• A hot cup of lower-sodium broth (vegetable, chicken, or beef) makes a great hunger-curbing midday snack when paired with a piece of reduced-fat cheese. You can keep the resealable boxes in the refrigerator at your office and heat a cup in the microwave.

• Being on the South Beach Diet doesn't mean that pasta can't still be a quick and satisfying meal for you when time is tight. Toss whole-wheat or spelt pasta with cooked flavored chicken strips, store-bought pesto, and skim-milk mozzarella; or fresh arugula, shrimp, and chopped canned tomatoes; or a few tablespoons of olive salad and chopped fresh basil; or chopped canned artichoke hearts, sliced sun-dried tomatoes, and freshly grated Parmesan.

• Make a quick, high-protein smoothie using 8 ounces low-fat, low-sugar soymilk, half a medium banana, 1 tablespoon sugar-free peanut butter, and 1 teaspoon granular sugar substitute.

• Wash and freeze fresh strawberries and blueberries on a tray or plate. Transfer to a freezer-proof bag or plastic container and pop them into your mouth when you need a refreshing fruity dessert. Great on a sweltering summer day—they'll evoke the flavor of natural frozen fruit pops. You can do the same thing with a medium-size banana.

• Toss marinated artichokes and pitted canned black olives with cooked whole-wheat or spelt pasta, extra-virgin olive oil, freshly ground black pepper, and salt. Since the artichokes are already marinated, you won't have to add extra spices or herbs. If you make the pasta ahead of time, all you have to do is combine the ingredients and then heat them in the microwave for dinner in mere minutes. You can also use canned tuna in place of pasta and add chopped tomato.

• For a high-protein twist on tuna salad, combine 2 (6-ounce) cans of water-packed tuna, 1 (15-ounce) can of rinsed and drained lentils, 1 chopped tomato, 2 chopped celery stalks, ⅓ cup of fresh lemon juice, 3 tablespoons of extra-virgin olive oil, 2 minced garlic cloves, and salt and freshly ground black pepper to taste. Makes 4 servings.

• Combine 2 (15-ounce) cans of split peas with 1 cup of water in a medium saucepan. Add 2 diced celery stalks, 1 diced carrot, 1 small diced onion, 2 minced garlic cloves, and a big pinch of salt and freshly ground black pepper; simmer until the vegetables are tender and the flavor is deep, 20 to 30 minutes. Adjust seasonings and serve hot. You can chop up a slice or two of boiled ham to sprinkle over the top, if you'd like.

• Purée ½ cup blueberries (or other berries) in a food processor. Fold into 1 cup whipped topping. Dollop 2 tablespoons of the topping over your favorite flavor of sugar-free gelatin (Phases 2 and 3).

• Steam broccoli until tender, top with low-fat cheddar cheese, and broil until the cheese is melted, about 2 minutes. Serve as a side dish.

• Using a food processor, shred celery root. Toss with shredded cole slaw mix, lemon juice, extra-virgin olive oil, and salt and freshly ground black pepper for a unique and tasty slaw.

• Season 4 (6-ounce) boneless, skinless chicken breasts with salt and pepper and toss with 2 tablespoons chopped chipotle in adobo sauce. Bake at 400°F until cooked through, about 20 minutes.

• Layer reduced-fat pepper Jack cheese, sliced avocado, and sliced tomato on half of a whole-wheat tortilla. Fold over and bake in the toaster oven at 325°F until the cheese is melted and the tortilla is lightly toasted, 5 to 10 minutes.

• Layer alternating slices of fresh tomato and skim-milk mozzarella; drizzle with extra-virgin olive oil and store-bought pesto. Sprinkle with salt and freshly ground black pepper.

• Place cooked Italian chicken strips in a microwave-safe baking dish; spoon sugar-free pasta sauce over the top and gently warm in the microwave. Top with thin slices of skim-milk mozzarella. Transfer the dish to the toaster oven or oven and bake at 375°F until the cheese is golden and bubbly, about 5 minutes. You can add thawed frozen spinach under the cheese before baking, if you'd like. Just squeeze out the excess liquid first.

• Cut cooked Southwest-flavored chicken strips into ¼-inch slices. Toss with torn lettuce, sliced canned hearts of palm, chopped tomatoes (canned or fresh), extra-virgin olive oil, low-fat or fat-free plain yogurt, fresh lemon juice, freshly ground black pepper, and salt for a quick ranch salad.

• Cut skim-milk mozzarella into ¼-inch cubes; toss with sliced sun-dried tomatoes and a bit of olive oil from the tomato jar (or with jarred olive salad), a pinch of Italian seasoning, and salt and freshly ground black pepper to taste. Serve alongside, or tossed into, a fresh green salad.

• For a risotto-style rice dish: In the microwave, heat leftover instant whole-grain brown rice with frozen peas, extra-virgin olive oil, Italian seasoning, and salt and freshly ground black pepper. Mix in freshly grated Parmesan cheese just before serving.

• For a quick snack or appetizer, make an avocado spread: Mash a ripe avocado, then mix in fresh salsa and a drop or two of hot sauce and salt to taste. Spread on whole-grain crackers.

• Make a quick bean mash by puréeing 1 (15-ounce) can of rinsed and drained Great Northern beans with 2 tablespoons of pesto. Add 4 to 6 cups of chicken stock to turn it into white bean soup!

Getting Ahead

Having part of your prep work done and ready to go or preparing "make-ahead and freeze" dishes when you have a little extra time will go a long way in helping you organize your South Beach Quick and Easy kitchen.

Start by taking time over the weekend to think about your meals for the week. Are you cooking for a family or just for yourself? Do you like to take lunches to school or to work? Would it be helpful to have breakfast ready to go in the morning, so you can fit in some exercise and then have time to eat before the day gets started? These are the kind of questions that I ask myself so that I can efficiently organize the kitchen to prepare tasty and nutritious meals.

Here are some of the things you can do to get ahead.

Think about items you can double up on in order to save prep time for multiple recipes. For example, if you like chicken, you could poach several pounds of skinless chicken breasts. Let the meat cool completely and then wrap and refrigerate it. Over the course of a few days, you'll have what you need to make several different chicken dishes, including Mexican Chicken Soup (page

120), Cajun Chicken Salad (page 194), Provolone Chicken Melts (page 267), or Peanut Chicken with Noodles (page 285). You'll only spend time preparing the chicken once, and then it will be freshly cooked and at your fingertips when you need it. You'll want to use chicken within 3 days of cooking, so keep that in mind as you plan.

If you plan a few meals in advance, you can easily chop up vegetables ahead of time. Generally, you can store ingredients that are added at the same time together. For example, if the onion, celery, and carrot for a soup are added to the pot at the same time, you can chop them ahead and place them together in a resealable plastic bag with the air pressed out or in an airtight container. When it comes time to cook, you'll add your prepared veggies to the pot all at once. This works best for dry vegetables (onions, carrots, celery, root vegetables); save the prep work on potatoes and moisture-rich vegetables, like tomatoes, for when you're ready to cook. You can cut vegetables up to 2 days ahead.

Double, triple, or even quadruple the recipe for our quick vinaigrettes (you find many that require just a few ingredients with the salad recipes in this book). Our vinaigrettes are easy to make and are free from the stabilizers and sugars you'll find in many store-bought brands. They'll keep for up to 2 weeks in the refrigerator—you can even store them in the same jar you use to make them! You'll be amazed at how satisfying it is to quickly throw together a salad when the fresh dressing is already on hand.

When you have extra time over the weekend, use it to prepare dishes and key ingredients that can be portioned and frozen. Then later in the week (or month!), all you have to do is defrost, heat, and serve. Good dishes to

Quick, Healthy Ways to Prepare Veggies

Looking for ways to cook your vegetables that are fast, easy, and healthy? I highly recommend steaming. The only equipment you need is a saucepan with a lid and a steamer insert. Try this technique with asparagus, green beans, broccoli, packaged mixed veggies, and more. Here are some simple steaming basics.

1. Place an inch or two of water and a steamer insert in a large saucepan, cover, and bring the water to a boil.

2. While the water is coming to a boil, prepare (peel or cut) your vegetables.

3. Place the vegetables in the basket and cover the pot.

4. Cook for a minute or two. Remember that the longer you steam, the less crunchy the vegetables will be—and they will become overcooked if steamed for too long.

5. Remove from the heat, drizzle with extra-virgin olive oil, sprinkle with salt and freshly ground black pepper, and serve with your favorite dishes.

A second quick and healthy way to prepare vegetables is in the microwave. Place the vegetables of your choice in a microwave-safe dish with 2 or 3 tablespoons of water and cover. During cooking, make sure the veggies are stirred or rotated. Depending on the type of vegetable, microwaving will take approximately 2 to 4 minutes per cup. For instance, 1 cup of broccoli or cauliflower takes 2 or 3 minutes; 1 cup of brussels sprouts, carrots, or green beans takes 3 or 4 minutes; and $\frac{1}{2}$ cup of sliced summer squash or zucchini is ready in about 3 or 4 minutes.

make ahead and freeze include Salmon Cakes (page 246), Rigatoni with Turkey Sausage and Mozzarella (page 256), Chicken Jambalaya (page 258), South Beach Chicken Paella (page 281), Chicken Pot Pie (page 302), Mini Greek Meatballs (page 322), Eggplant Bulgur Lasagna (page 409), and Quinoa Pilaf (page 418). Some dishes need spices adjusted after thawing and reheating. If so, you may need an extra sprinkle of salt, freshly ground pepper, or fresh or dried herbs.

You can also make, portion, and freeze rice and grains ahead (they'll keep for up to 3 months in the freezer). Do the same with the filling for Veggie Burrito (page 380).

Soups, stews, and chili freeze beautifully, too. Be sure to cool food to room temperature before freezing (see freezing tips on page 70).

Freezing isn't just for savory foods; you can also make and freeze desserts ahead of time so you'll have them ready when the holiday frenzy strikes or in case guests drop by unannounced. Portioning and freezing desserts will also help you from overdoing it on sweets, especially if you are cooking for just yourself or for a small family. Peanut Butter and Jelly Cookies (page 453), Flourless Chocolate-Raspberry Cakes (page 462), and Orange Poppy Seed Cupcakes (page 468) all freeze well. Any special freezing instructions for these dishes are noted with the recipe.

Food Safety

Refrigerating and freezing foods keeps them both fresh and safe. There are many important food safety guidelines to follow (look to special supermarket pamphlets and food safety Web sites for more information). Here are some basic tips to get you started.

- Set your refrigerator at a temperature of 40°F or below; keep a refrigerator thermometer in your unit so you can check it periodically. You may find you need to set it lower in the summer than you do in the winter. Adjust the temperature up or down by a few degrees if you find items like lettuce or milk are either freezing or are not cold enough.
- Clean the fridge regularly to keep it free from bacteria that can easily pass to fresh foods.
- Keep fresh meats, poultry, and fish in the coldest part of the refrigerator and use them within 2 or 3 days of purchase.
- Keep eggs safe from damage, moisture loss, and odor absorption by keeping them in the refrigerator in their original containers, not in the egg cups on the refrigerator door. Eggs are freshest within 1 week from the date on the carton but will keep for a total of 4 to 5 weeks. Egg whites can be refrigerated for up to 4 days or frozen in an airtight container for up to 6 months. Thaw frozen whites in the refrigerator before using.

Proper use of the freezer will help you keep foods safe and better organize your South Beach Quick and Easy kitchen. Here are some general freezing rules.

• Make sure your freezer is at 0°F or just below (keep a freezer thermometer in the freezer to monitor the temperature).

10 Kitchen Tools That Make Any Meal Quicker

With the right equipment, cooking becomes a whole lot easier—and more fun. Save time and effort with the following essential items.

1. Food processor or blender. A food processor is great for chopping, slicing, and shredding vegetables as well as chopping nuts, mincing garlic, and making doughs and pie crusts. Blenders are best for quickly combining liquid items, such as soups, sauces, and dressings. Hand blenders make for quick and easy cleanup if you make a lot of puréed soups.

2. Nonstick skillets. No one wants to spend hours cleaning grease-coated pans. Nonstick skillets (it's good to have both large and small) are terrific for cooking both meat and egg dishes.

3. Steamer basket. Use this tool for steaming vegetables, chicken, and fish.

4. A good set of knives. High-quality knives help you slice and dice quickly and easily; keep them sharp and out of children's reach.

5. A good set of measuring cups and spoons. You'll need to have glass measuring cups for liquid ingredients, metal or plastic measuring cups for dry ingredients, and measuring spoons handy nearly every time you cook.

• Always label and date food items (using freezer tape and a permanent marker) before storing them in the freezer. This will help you keep track of what you have on hand and ensure that you use it within a month or two.

• Freeze foods in specially designed freezer containers, heavy-duty aluminum foil, and freezer-weight resealable plastic bags. Do not use regular foil, plastic wrap, or

6. Toaster oven. If you're cooking for one, consider using the toaster oven in lieu of the large oven; it heats up quickly and is great for baking, roasting, and broiling.

7. Freezer-proof plastic storage containers and storage bags. Use these to store foods you prepare in advance in the fridge and the freezer. They're also handy to transport lunches to work or school.

8. Microplane or box grater. You'll use these for grating fresh Parmesan and other hard cheeses. Microplane graters are also perfect for quickly and efficiently zesting citrus fruits and grating whole nutmeg, fresh ginger, fresh coconut, and chocolate.

9. Kitchen timer. Purchase one or two small digital timers. If you have more than one, you can mark each individually when simultaneously using them for different dishes (mark pieces of first-aid tape or masking tape with a permanent marker and lightly affix to each timer).

10. Permanent marker and a roll of freezer or masking tape. You'll want to label and date all the ingredients and foods that you prepare ahead and put in the freezer for later use. This will help keep you organized, and you'll find you waste less food when the contents and dates are easily visible. If you're using plastic freezer bags, you can simply write on the bags; when using freezer-proof plastic containers, mark the tape and affix it to your containers. When you are finished with the contents, simply clean the tape off and repeat the process.

plastic bags for freezer storage, as they are not vapor- or moisture-proof.

- Always press the air out of plastic freezer bags before sealing.
- Allow an inch or two of space in plastic containers of soup or other liquid ingredients that you want to freeze. These items will expand into the empty space as they freeze.
- Never refreeze meats, poultry, and seafood or cooked defrosted foods. The taste will be compromised and you'll also risk bacterial growth.
- Use the microwave to defrost frozen foods or thaw them in the refrigerator. For safety's sake, never thaw frozen foods at room temperature.

Now that you've organized your kitchen and perhaps learned a few new things about cooking and eating healthy foods, you're ready to dive into a new world of delicious South Beach Quick and Easy recipes. We hope you enjoy!

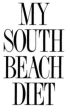

MY SOUTH BEACH DIET

It's a big advantage for us to be on the South Beach Diet together.

After hearing about Dr. Agatston's approach to healthy eating on a Pittsburgh TV news program, my husband, Tim, and I decided to give the South Beach Diet a try. The idea of eating the right carbs and the right fats made a lot of sense to us, and we especially trusted Dr. Agatston since he was a renowned cardiologist. Our weight has been an issue most of our adult lives, and while we had tried other diet plans in the past (like Weight Watchers), none of them worked as fast or felt like as much of a "lifestyle" change as the South Beach Diet. We each lost 60 pounds within 7 months. Not only did we notice the difference in our appearance, but our health conditions also improved. With our lower blood pressure and cholesterol, we were feeling better, too!

It's a big advantage for us to be on the South Beach Diet together. We encourage and coach each other along the way. My husband even shares in the cooking; he makes a great rainbow trout with wine and caper sauce! We also both agree that our success was due to a few key things. First, our cupboards were always fully stocked with all the ingredients needed for trying a variety of recipes from the original *South Beach Diet Cookbook*. Second, we always kept good snacks around—like nuts and reduced-fat cheese—and we made sure to take our fish oil supplements. Third, we added exercise to our plan by investing in a treadmill. We both walk from half hour to an hour, three or four times a week. To build up muscle, which is especially important for women, we also started working with hand weights and resistance-training exercises.

We have had our share of setbacks, especially during the holidays when it's hard to resist specially prepared foods. But we've learned from our mistakes and realize we can go back to Phase 1 at any point. I've also found it very useful to go back and reread *The South Beach Diet* book, which I've done three times!

Our family and friends are extremely encouraged by our weight loss. We have even managed to convince a few of them to start the diet, too! This is how we plan to live out the rest of our lives, and we will forever be grateful to Dr. Agatston and his staff for teaching us to eat better and live better.

—GINA AND TIM P., TORONTO, OHIO

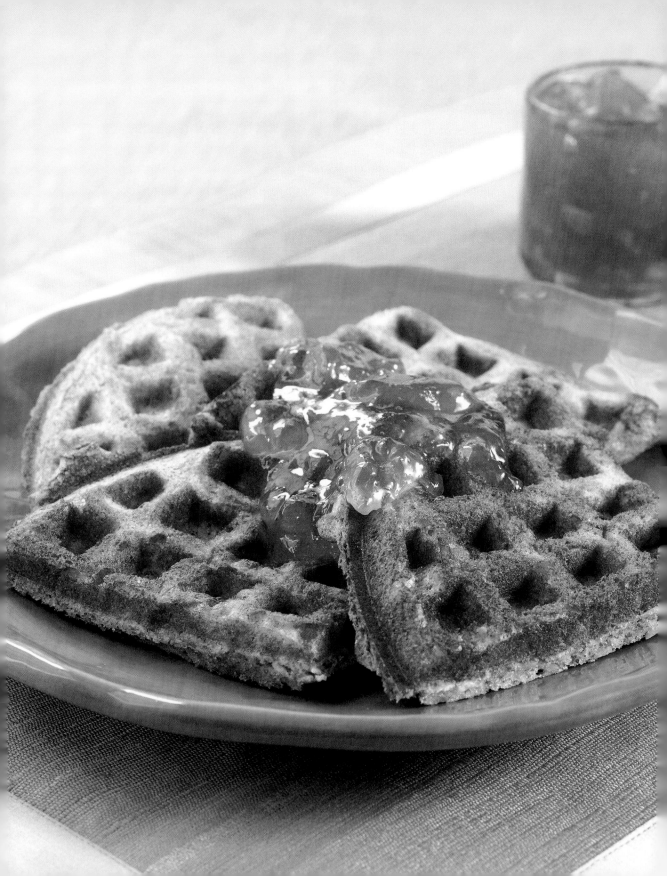

BREAKFAST

Think of eating breakfast as the beginning of a journey. Common sense dictates that you should fill your tank before you hit the road: The same applies when you're preparing your body for the day ahead. Fueling up with protein-rich foods and good fats like eggs, cheeses, and lean meats, as well as high-fiber vegetables and fruits, will not only provide you with the energy you need to start the day but will also satisfy you from early to mid morning.

In the coming pages you'll find delicious options—like Smoked Salmon Scramble, Papaya Parfait, Almond Energy Blast, and South Beach Eggsadilla—that can be prepared in 10 minutes or less. You won't miss goodies like pancakes, waffles, and muffins because they're included, filled with heart-healthy whole-grain and buckwheat flours, oats, blueberries, and pears.

◄*Buttermilk Waffles with Jam (page 76)*

Buttermilk Waffles with Jam

PREP TIME: 10 minutes

COOK TIME: 5 minutes per waffle (depending on size
            of waffle iron)

A warm waffle topped with your favorite jam makes a hearty and special breakfast anytime. Once prepared, these can be wrapped individually and frozen for up to 3 weeks. Reheat in the toaster, using low heat, until warmed through.

1 cup whole-wheat flour

1 cup old-fashioned rolled oats

1 tablespoon plus 1 teaspoon baking powder

3 tablespoons granular sugar substitute

3 tablespoons canola oil

1¼ cups 1 percent or fat-free buttermilk

½ cup water

1 large egg

¾ cup sugar-free jam, any flavor

Combine flour, oats, baking powder, salt, and sugar substitute in a medium bowl. Whisk together oil, buttermilk, water, and egg in a separate bowl. Pour the buttermilk mixture into the flour mixture and stir until combined.

Heat waffle iron; coat lightly with cooking spray. Add a generous ½ cup batter per waffle and cook until browned and crisp, about 5 minutes. Dollop with jam and serve.

Makes 4 (1 waffle) servings

NUTRITION AT A GLANCE

Per serving: 360 calories, 15 g fat, 2.5 g saturated fat, 11 g protein, 56 g carbohydrate, 6 g dietary fiber, 490 mg sodium

Breakfast Turkey Stack

PREP TIME: 5 minutes   **COOK TIME:** 15 minutes

Quick homemade turkey patties piled high with juicy tomatoes and bubbly melted cheese make an irresistible breakfast stack that offers a change of pace from the usual eggs and toast. Pair with a salad for a great brunch or lunch. Patties can be individually wrapped and frozen for up to 1 month; just defrost and simply reheat in the oven or microwave.

- 1 pound ground turkey breast
- 4 teaspoons sugar-free pancake syrup
- ½ teaspoon dried sage
- ¼ teaspoon cayenne pepper
- ¼ teaspoon salt
- ⅛ teaspoon freshly ground black pepper
- ⅛ teaspoon ground ginger
- 1 teaspoon extra-virgin olive oil
- 1 large beefsteak tomato, cut into 4 slices
- 4 (1-ounce) slices reduced-fat cheddar cheese

Heat oven to broil.

Combine turkey, syrup, sage, cayenne, salt, pepper, and ginger in a mixing bowl and mix well. Divide into 4 (½-inch-thick) patties.

Heat oil in a large nonstick skillet over medium-high heat; cook patties until well browned and cooked through, about 4 minutes per side. Remove from heat.

Lay tomato slices in a single layer in a baking dish; season with salt and pepper. Top each slice with 1 turkey patty and 1 cheese slice; broil until cheese is melted, about 2 minutes. Serve hot.

Makes 4 servings

NUTRITION AT A GLANCE

Per serving: 220 calories, 7 g fat, 3.5 g saturated fat, 36 g protein, 4 g carbohydrate, 0 g dietary fiber, 380 mg sodium

Swiss Cheese and Vegetable Omelet

PREP TIME: 10 minutes   **COOK TIME:** 8 minutes

The key to easy omelet making is a nonstick pan, which allows you to use a minimum amount of oil and still be able to keep the eggs from sticking or overcooking. Omelets cook quickly, so be sure to have all of your ingredients ready before you start.

- 2 teaspoons extra-virgin olive oil, divided
- ½ small onion, thinly sliced
- ½ bell pepper, any color, cut into ¼-inch squares
- 1 small plum tomato, diced
- ¼ teaspoon Italian seasoning or dried basil
- 3 eggs, lightly beaten
- ¼ teaspoon salt

  Pinch ground black pepper

- 1 ounce reduced-fat Swiss cheese, finely grated (¼ cup)

Heat 1 teaspoon of the oil in a large nonstick skillet over medium heat. Add onion and cook until softened, about 3 minutes. Add bell pepper, tomato, and Italian seasoning; cook 3 minutes more. Transfer vegetables to a plate.

Season eggs with salt and pepper. Heat remaining oil in the same skillet over medium heat, add eggs, and let set for 30 seconds. Using a heatproof spatula, gently lift edges of eggs while tilting pan to allow uncooked eggs to run underneath until eggs are set, about 1 minute. Sprinkle cheese and vegetables over half of omelet. Fold omelet over filling, slide onto a plate, cut in half, and serve.

Makes 2 servings

NUTRITION AT A GLANCE

Per serving: 220 calories, 15 g fat, 3.5 g saturated fat, 14 g protein, 7 g carbohydrate, 1 g dietary fiber, 430 mg sodium

Blueberry Buckwheat Pancakes

PREP TIME: 10 minutes

COOK TIME: About 4 to 6 minutes per serving

Tangy buttermilk adds extra rise to these cakey, fruit-filled pancakes, and buckwheat—high in iron and low in gluten—gives them a delicious toasted flavor. Top with sugar-free pancake syrup or low-fat or fat-free yogurt.

½ cup buckwheat flour

½ cup whole-grain pastry flour

2 teaspoons granular sugar substitute

1 teaspoon baking soda

1 cup 1 percent or fat-free buttermilk

2 large eggs, lightly beaten

¼ cup trans-fat-free margarine, melted

1¼ cups blueberries

Heat oven to 200°F.

Combine buckwheat flour, pastry flour, sugar substitute, baking soda, and salt in a mixing bowl. Combine buttermilk, eggs, and margarine in another mixing bowl. Add wet mixture to dry mixture and stir just until combined well, being careful not to overmix. Stir in blueberries.

Heat griddle over medium heat until hot enough to cause drops of water to scatter over the surface, about 3 minutes; lightly coat with cooking spray. Spoon batter onto griddle to form 3-inch rounds; cook until golden on both sides, 2 to 3 minutes per side. Transfer to a heatproof platter and place in the oven to keep warm until ready to serve.

Makes 4 servings (4 pancakes per serving)

NUTRITION AT A GLANCE

Per serving: 260 calories, 13 g fat, 4 g saturated fat, 9 g protein, 27 g carbohydrate, 4 g dietary fiber, 500 mg sodium

Savory Egg, Ham, and Cheese Crêpes

PREP TIME: 20 minutes (includes time to let batter rest)
COOK TIME: 25 minutes

If a wheat or gluten allergy won't usually allow you to enjoy crepes, then this delicious breakfast dish is for you! Chickpea flour—a nonwheat, gluten-free flour made from ground dried chickpeas—creates filling protein-, and iron-rich crepes that are just as tasty as they are nutritious. Look for the flour in your health food store. If you have some fresh herbs on hand, add a chopped tablespoon or two just before rolling up the crêpes.

Crêpe Batter:

⅓ cup chickpea flour

⅓ cup 1 percent milk

1 tablespoon plus 1½ teaspoons warm water

1 large egg

1 tablespoon plus 1½ teaspoons canola oil

⅛ teaspoon freshly ground black pepper

Crêpes:

2 teaspoons canola oil, divided

4 (1-ounce) slices low-fat, low-sodium boiled or smoked ham (not honey glazed)

4 (¾-ounce) slices reduced-fat Swiss cheese

4 large eggs, lightly beaten

Salt and freshly ground black pepper

For the crêpe batter: Purée flour, milk, water, egg, oil, salt, and pepper in a blender until smooth, about 1 minute. Set aside to rest for 15 minutes.

For the crêpes: Heat 1 teaspoon of the oil in an 8-inch nonstick skillet or crêpe pan over medium heat. Add 2 tablespoons of the batter, tilting the pan so that batter forms a thin layer. Cook until edges begin to brown, about 1 minute. Carefully flip the crêpe over and cook until golden on the bottom, about 1 more minute. Transfer crêpe, golden side down, to a plate. Without adding any additional oil, repeat with remaining batter, stacking crêpes, to make all 4 crêpes.

Lay each crêpe, golden side down, on a serving plate. Top each with 1 ham slice and 1 cheese slice.

Season eggs with salt and pepper. Heat remaining oil in a nonstick skillet over medium-high heat. Add eggs and stir occasionally until set, about 2 minutes. Divide eggs among prepared crêpes, roll up, and serve.

Makes 4 servings

NUTRITION AT A GLANCE

Per serving: 270 calories, 16 g fat, 3.5 g saturated fat, 20 g protein, 9 g carbohydrate, 1 g dietary fiber, 530 mg sodium

Mango Smoothie

PREP TIME: 10 minutes

With just a few ingredients, you can whip up this luscious fruit smoothie. The natural sugars and fibrous nature of mangoes make a rich and filling breakfast drink.

2 mangoes, peeled, pitted, and diced

1½ cups sugar-free vanilla fat-free or low-fat yogurt

Ice cubes

Purée mangoes in blender. Add yogurt and 4 or 5 ice cubes; blend until thick and smooth, about 30 seconds. Pour into glasses and serve.

Makes 4 (1-cup) servings

NUTRITION AT A GLANCE

Per serving: 140 calories, 0 g fat, 0 g saturated fat, 4 g protein, 30 g carbohydrate, 1 g dietary fiber, 50 mg sodium

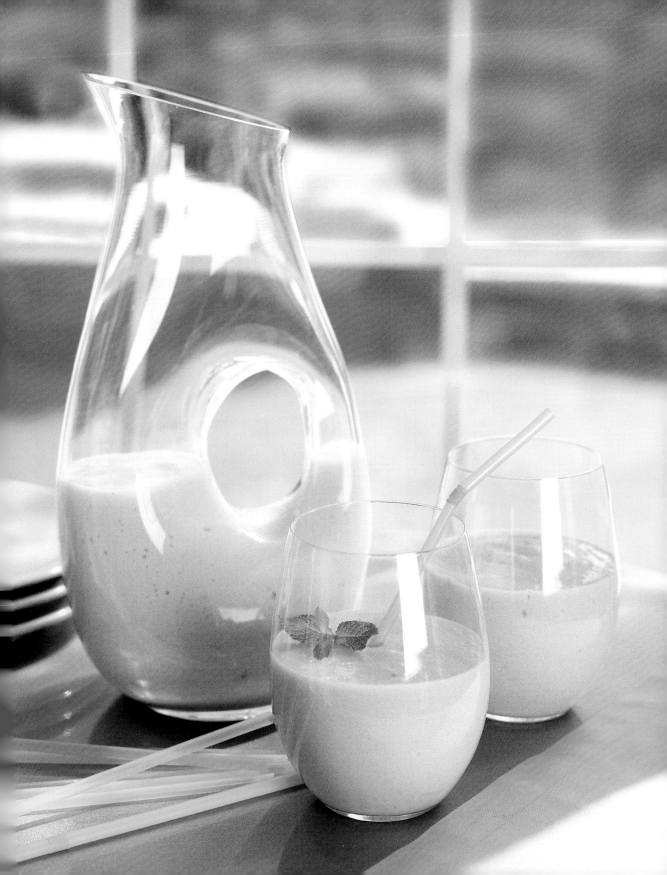

Spiced Oatmeal with Dried Apricot and Walnuts

PREP TIME: 5 minutes   **COOK TIME:** 20 minutes

This quick, heavenly oatmeal is made with steel-cut oats, a South Beach favorite because of their distinctive dense texture and high levels of protein, iron, and soluble fiber— satisfying nutrients that help boost energy. Make a double batch if you'd like; the oatmeal keeps for up to 5 days in the refrigerator.

¼ cup walnuts

2 cups water

½ cup steel-cut oats

12 dried apricots, cut into ¼-inch pieces

1½ teaspoons sugar-free pancake syrup

½ teaspoon ground cinnamon

Salt

Heat oven or toaster oven to 275°F. Spread walnuts on a baking tray and bake until fragrant and toasted, 8 to 10 minutes. Roughly chop.

MICROWAVE INSTRUCTIONS: While the nuts are toasting, combine water, oats, apricots, syrup, cinnamon, and a pinch of salt in an 8-cup microwave-safe bowl (the size of the bowl is important as it must allow the oats to bubble up without spilling over). Cover with plastic wrap, vent, and cook at full power for 5 to 7 minutes. Stir, replace plastic wrap, and cook for an additional 5 to 7 minutes, until liquid is mostly absorbed. Sprinkle with nuts and serve.

STOVETOP INSTRUCTIONS: Combine water and oats in a medium saucepan; soak overnight. Add apricots, syrup, and salt and bring to a boil over medium heat. Reduce heat and simmer, stirring occasionally, until liquid is mostly absorbed, 15 to 20 minutes. Sprinkle each serving with nuts and cinnamon.

Makes 4 (½-cup) servings

NUTRITION AT A GLANCE

Per serving: 180 calories, 6 g fat, ½ g saturated fat, 5 g protein, 28 g carbohydrate, 4 g dietary fiber, 80 mg sodium

Spicy Tomatillo Scramble

PREP TIME: 5 minutes   **COOK TIME: 8 minutes**

Tomatillos look like little green tomatoes, except that they have a delicate, husk-like covering and a sticky skin underneath. Slip the covering right off with your fingers and simply rinse the skin under tap water—you'll then have a delicious and tangy ingredient that can be diced and added to salsa, guacamole, Southwestern-style salads, or . . . scrambled eggs! Try this dish with a sprinkle of reduced-fat cheddar cheese, if desired, or scoop it into a whole-wheat tortilla in later phases.

- 2½ teaspoons canola oil, divided
- 1 medium tomatillo, papery skin removed and chopped into ¼-inch dice
- ½ small onion, diced
- 3 large eggs, lightly beaten
- 2 tablespoons medium-hot salsa
- Salt and freshly ground black pepper

Heat 1½ teaspoons of the oil in a medium skillet over medium-high heat. Add tomatillo and onion. Reduce heat to medium and cook, stirring frequently, until vegetables are softened and lightly browned, about 4 minutes. Remove vegetables from skillet.

Heat remaining oil in the same skillet over medium heat; add eggs, reduce heat to low, and allow eggs to set, 2 minutes. Sprinkle vegetables over eggs, season with a pinch of salt and pepper, and scramble until just cooked, about 1 minute more. Serve with salsa.

Makes 2 servings

NUTRITION AT A GLANCE

Per serving: 190 calories, 13 g fat, 3 g saturated fat, 10 g protein, 5 g carbohydrate, 0 g dietary fiber, 350 mg sodium

Almond Energy Blast

PREP TIME: 5 minutes

You'll go nuts for this creamy drink. Fresh almonds, along with silken tofu, yogurt, and soymilk, offer a satiating punch of protein that will help you power through the morning; it whips up quickly and travels well in a thermos for breakfast on the go. Silken tofu, available at health food stores and many supermarkets, is great for shakes and smoothies because of its smooth texture. WestSoy Soy Slender is a low-sugar brand we recommend.

> 1 cup low-fat, low-sugar vanilla soymilk
>
> ¾ cup plain fat-free or low-fat yogurt
>
> 6 ounces firm silken tofu
>
> ¼ cup dry-roasted almonds

Place soymilk, yogurt, tofu, and almonds in a blender. Blend until smooth, about 1 minute. Serve cold.

Makes 2 (1-cup) servings

NUTRITION AT A GLANCE

Per serving: 250 calories, 12 g fat, 1 g saturated fat, 15 g protein, 22 g carbohydrate, 2 g dietary fiber, 130 mg sodium

South Beach Eggsadilla

PREP TIME: 5 minutes   COOK TIME: 5 minutes

Quick enough for a weekday morning yet fun enough for a lazy Saturday, this Tex-Mex breakfast dish will get you off to a satisfying start. Add a spoonful of salsa if you like.

1 teaspoon extra-virgin olive oil

3 large eggs, lightly beaten

1 (8-inch) whole-wheat tortilla

2 ounces reduced-fat pepper Jack cheese, sliced

Salt and freshly ground black pepper

Heat oil in a large nonstick skillet over medium-high heat. Add eggs, reduce heat to medium, and scramble until cooked but still moist, about 2 minutes. Remove to a plate and season with salt and pepper.

Carefully wipe the pan with a paper towel. Replace on heat. Add tortilla and cook on both sides until warmed through, about 1 minute.

Leaving tortilla in the pan, top half of it with cheese and then with eggs; fold the other half over to form a quesadilla.

Cook on both sides until heated through, 1 minute more. Transfer to a cutting board, cut in half, and serve.

Makes 2 servings

NUTRITION AT A GLANCE

Per serving: 280 calories, 17 g fat, 7 g saturated fat, 18 g protein, 13 g carbohydrate, 1 g dietary fiber, 580 mg sodium

Yogurt with Apple-Prune Compote

PREP TIME: 5 minutes   COOK TIME: 20 minutes

We won't be surprised if our heart-healthy, fiber-rich compote becomes your new favorite yogurt topping. In addition to a tasty breakfast, this recipe also makes a nice snack or dessert. Serve the compote warm, cold, or at room temperature; you can also try it as a spread for whole-grain toast.

- 1 firm, sweet or semisweet apple (such as Fuji, Gala, Jonathan, or Golden Delicious), peeled, cored, and cut into ½-inch chunks
- ¾ cup pitted prunes, quartered
- 1 cup water
- 1 tablespoon orange juice
- 24 ounces plain fat-free or low-fat yogurt

Place apple, prunes, water, and juice in a small saucepan and bring to a boil. Reduce to a simmer and cook until prunes soften, about 10 minutes. Cool 5 minutes, then serve warm over yogurt. Store leftover compote in the refrigerator for up to 2 weeks.

Makes 6 servings

NUTRITION AT A GLANCE

Per serving: 110 calories, 1.5 g fat, 1 g saturated fat, 6 g protein, 20 g carbohydrate, 2 g dietary fiber, 75 mg sodium

Dutch Apple Pancake

PREP TIME: 10 minutes   **COOK TIME:** 25 minutes

This puffy, Dutch-style pancake is served piping hot, right from the skillet! We used a 10-inch pan to make ours, but if yours is smaller or larger, adjust the cooking time slightly (shorter if the pan is bigger; longer if it's smaller) to accommodate.

- 2 tablespoons trans-fat-free margarine, melted, divided
- 1 medium Granny Smith apple, peeled, cored, and cut into ½-inch slices
- ⅓ cup whole-grain pastry flour
- 2 tablespoons sugar
- 1 tablespoon granular sugar substitute
- ½ teaspoon ground cinnamon
- ¼ teaspoon ground nutmeg
- ¾ cup 1 percent milk
- 4 eggs, lightly beaten

Heat oven to 400°F.

Heat 1 tablespoon of the margarine in a large cast-iron skillet over medium heat. Add apple and cook until softened and lightly browned, about 5 minutes.

Purée remaining margarine, flour, sugar, sugar substitute, cinnamon, nutmeg, milk, and eggs in a blender until just combined, about 1 minute. Pour batter into skillet, over apples. Bake until puffed and set, about 15 minutes. Serve hot.

Makes 4 servings

NUTRITION AT A GLANCE

Per serving: 210 calories, 10 g fat, 3 g saturated fat, 9 g protein, 21 g carbohydrate, 2 g dietary fiber, 140 mg sodium

Smoked Salmon Scramble

PREP TIME: 5 minutes   **COOK TIME:** 5 minutes

Smoked salmon and smooth cream cheese are a classic pair, but wait until you try them warm and melted into freshly scrambled eggs—what a way to start the day!

- 1 teaspoon canola oil
- 3 large eggs (or 2 large eggs and 2 large egg whites), lightly beaten
- 1 ounce smoked salmon, cut into thin strips
- 1 ounce reduced-fat cream cheese, cut into ¼-inch pieces
- 1 tablespoon finely chopped fresh chives
- Freshly ground black pepper (optional)

Heat oil in a nonstick skillet over medium-high heat for 1 to 2 minutes. Add eggs and allow to set, 10 seconds. Sprinkle salmon, cream cheese, and chives over eggs. Scramble until just cooked, about 1 minute, being careful not to overcook. Season to taste with pepper, if desired. Serve hot.

Makes 2 servings

NUTRITION AT A GLANCE

Per serving: 170 calories, 12 g fat, 3 g saturated fat, 14 g protein, 1 g carbohydrate, 0 g dietary fiber, 160 mg sodium

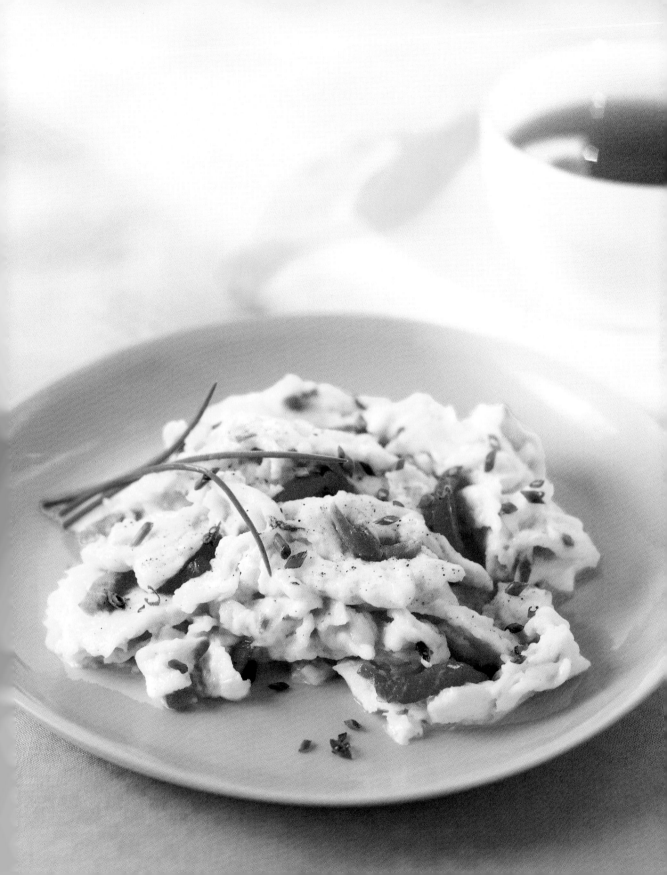

Turkey Hash

PREP TIME: 10 minutes   **COOK TIME: 20 minutes**

You don't have to give up this breakfast favorite on South Beach; slightly modified with sweet turnips and turkey breast, our modern interpretation is delicious. Try it topped with a poached egg.

> 2 teaspoons extra-virgin olive oil
>
> 1 small onion, chopped
>
> 1 small red bell pepper, diced
>
> 2 medium turnips, peeled and cut into ½-inch dice
>
> ½ teaspoon dried thyme
>
> 1 pound cooked skinless roast turkey breast, cut into ¼-inch cubes
>
> ¼ cup fat-free half-and-half
>
> Salt and freshly ground black pepper

Heat oil in a large nonstick skillet over medium heat. Add onion and bell pepper and cook until softened, about 3 minutes. Add turnips and thyme; stir and cook until tender, about 10 minutes. Stir in turkey and half-and-half; simmer until liquid has thickened slightly, about 3 minutes. Season with salt and pepper to taste.

Makes 8 (¹/₂-cup) servings

NUTRITION AT A GLANCE

Per serving: 110 calories, 2 g fat, 0 g saturated fat, 18 g protein, 4 g carbohydrate, 1 g dietary fiber, 100 mg sodium

Egg, Bacon, and Tomato "Sandwiches"

PREP TIME: 5 minutes   COOK TIME: 15 minutes

Oven-baked tomatoes, smoky Canadian bacon, and a touch of mustard make an outstanding breadless, low-fat twist on eggs Benedict. A little vinegar is the simple secret to a perfect poached egg.

- 2 medium tomatoes, each cut into 4 slices
- 2 teaspoons Dijon mustard
- 1 tablespoon chopped fresh tarragon (optional)
- 4 (1-ounce) slices Canadian bacon
- 1 tablespoon white vinegar
- 4 large eggs
- Salt and freshly ground black pepper

Heat oven to 400°F.

Season tomato slices with salt and pepper; place 4 of them in a single layer in a nonreactive baking dish, spread with mustard, and sprinkle with tarragon, if using.

Cook bacon in a large skillet over medium heat until lightly browned, about 2 minutes per side. Lay 1 bacon slice over each mustard-spread tomato slice. Transfer to the oven and bake until tomatoes begin to bubble, about 10 minutes.

Fill a straight-sided skillet or wide saucepan with 2 inches of water. Add vinegar and bring to a gentle simmer. Crack each egg into a separate cup or bowl. Carefully slide each egg into the just-simmering water. Cook until desired doneness, about 3 minutes for soft-centered; remove with a slotted spoon, placing 1 egg atop each bacon slice. Top with remaining tomato slices and serve.

Makes 4 servings

NUTRITION AT A GLANCE

Per serving: 140 calories, 7 g fat, 2 g saturated fat, 13 g protein, 7 g carbohydrate, 0 g dietary fiber, 580 mg sodium

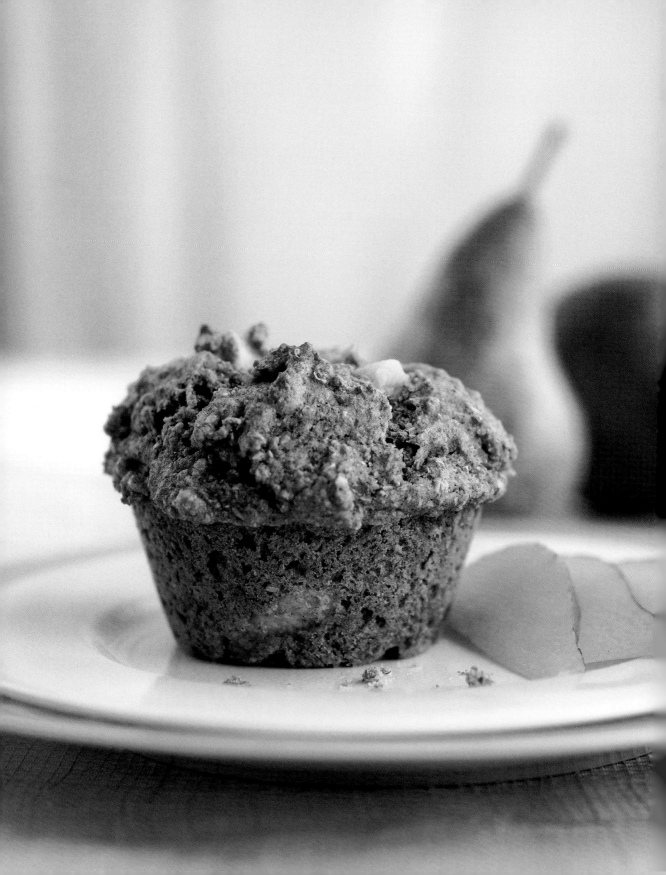

Pear Bran Muffins

PREP TIME: 15 minutes   **COOK TIME: 20 minutes**

These wholesome, satisfying muffins are filled with tender pieces of pear and spiced with cinnamon. They freeze well; just heat in the toaster or microwave before serving.

  1½ cups whole-grain pastry flour

    1 cup wheat bran

    2 tablespoons granular sugar substitute

  1¼ teaspoons ground cinnamon

  1¼ teaspoons baking soda

   ¼ teaspoon salt

  1¼ cups 1 percent or fat-free buttermilk

    2 large eggs, lightly beaten

    3 tablespoons canola oil

    1 Bosc pear, cored and cut into ¼-inch dice

  1½ teaspoons vanilla extract

Heat oven to 350°F. Line a muffin tin with paper liners or lightly coat with cooking spray.

Combine flour, bran, sugar substitute, cinnamon, baking soda, and salt in a large mixing bowl. Combine buttermilk, eggs, oil, pear, and vanilla in another mixing bowl.

Make a well in the center of the dry ingredients. Add wet ingredients to dry ingredients and mix just to combine; do not overmix. Divide batter evenly into muffin cups. Bake for 20 minutes. Cool and serve.

Makes 12 servings

NUTRITION AT A GLANCE

Per serving: 130 calories, 5 g fat, ½ g saturated fat, 5 g protein, 20 g carbohydrate, 5 g dietary fiber, 200 mg sodium

Papaya Parfait

PREP TIME: 10 minutes

This refreshing, pretty parfait will get you up and running in the morning.

½ cup cubed papaya

¼ teaspoon fresh lime juice

1 cup vanilla fat-free or low-fat yogurt, divided

½ cup multigrain, low-sugar breakfast cereal, divided

Toss papaya with lime juice. Layer ¼ cup yogurt, 2 tablespoons cereal, ¼ cup papaya, another ¼ cup yogurt, and another 2 tablespoons cereal in a glass dessert cup or bowl. Repeat with remaining ingredients in another cup. Serve immediately.

Makes 2 servings

NUTRITION AT A GLANCE

Per serving: 110 calories, .5 g fat, 0 g saturated fat, 6 g protein, 21 g carbohydrate, 2 g dietary fiber, 115 mg sodium

Southwest-Style Chicken Frittata

PREP TIME: 5 minutes　　　**COOK TIME: 10 minutes**

This yummy egg dish comes out of the oven puffed up and steaming, with edges crisp and golden. If you don't have leftover chicken, season and cook a 6- to 8-ounce boneless breast on a grill pan over medium-high heat, 5 to 6 minutes per side. Leftover frittata keeps in the fridge for 2 days and easily reheats in a low oven or microwave. We used an 8-inch pan, but if your pan is larger, just cook the frittata for 2 or 3 minutes less.

- 6 large eggs, lightly beaten
- 1 (6-ounce) boneless, skinless chicken breast, cooked and thinly sliced
- 2 ounces shredded reduced-fat cheddar cheese (½ cup)
- ½ cup salsa

  Salt and freshly ground black pepper

Heat broiler. Season eggs with salt and pepper.

Heat an 8-inch cast-iron or ovenproof nonstick skillet over medium heat. Spray pan (including sides) with cooking spray and add chicken, dispersing meat around the pan in a single layer.

Pour eggs over chicken and cook, undisturbed, until eggs are almost set, about 5 minutes.

Sprinkle eggs evenly with cheese and dollop with salsa. Broil until eggs are set, frittata is puffed up, and cheese is melted, about 1 minute. Cut into 4 portions and serve hot.

Makes 4 servings

NUTRITION AT A GLANCE

Per serving: 200 calories, 10 g fat, 4 g saturated fat, 23 g protein, 3 g carbohydrate, 0 g dietary fiber, 430 mg sodium

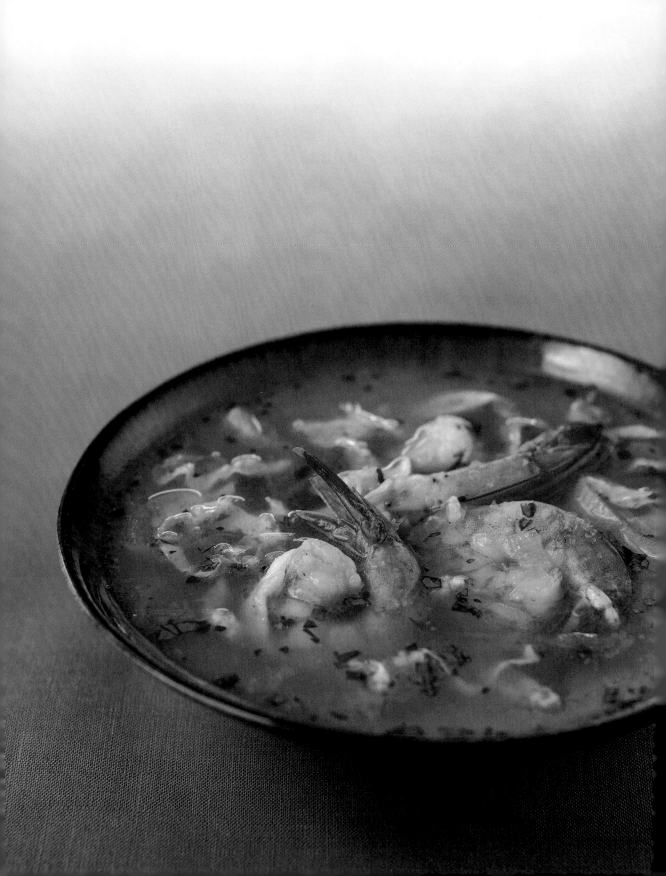

SOUPS AND SNACKS

A few pantry staples, like lower-sodium broths, dried spices, fresh garlic, and canned tomatoes and beans, plus a couple of vegetables and perhaps some meat or fish, will allow you to quickly assemble a wide array of fantastic soups. Mexican Chicken Soup, Curried Zucchini Soup, and Shrimp Gazpacho are just some of the ones you'll find here.

Since soups freeze beautifully, try making them ahead when you have a little extra time—you can even freeze and store them in portion-size containers, which later become an instant portable option for the office or for school.

Many of the nutritious snacks in this chapter can also be prepared in advance and travel well, too, so you can nibble on them in the car or at your desk when midday hunger strikes. Favorites like Warm Artichoke Dip are also great for entertaining.

◄ *Thai Shrimp Soup with Lime and Cilantro (page 112)*

Thai Shrimp Soup with Lime and Cilantro

PREP TIME: 15 minutes   **COOK TIME:** 12 minutes

Keep one or two Asian basics (like fish sauce) in your pantry and, with the addition of some fresh lime and ginger, you'll be amazed at how easy it is to whip up a host of vibrant, one-pot dishes like this delicious spicy soup. For a heartier version, add cooked soba noodles in later phases. Top with chopped scallion in place of cilantro, if you'd like.

- 1 tablespoon canola oil
- 3 tablespoons minced fresh ginger
- 1 small onion, thinly sliced
- 5 cups lower-sodium chicken broth
- ¼ teaspoon red pepper flakes
- 1 (½-pound) head napa cabbage, thinly sliced (about 3 cups)
- 1½ pounds fresh or thawed frozen shrimp, peeled and deveined
- 2 tablespoons Asian fish sauce (see page 27)
- 2 teaspoons grated lime zest
- ¼ cup fresh lime juice
- ½ cup chopped fresh cilantro (optional)

Heat oil in a large saucepan over medium heat. Add ginger and onion; cook, stirring often, until fragrant, about 3 minutes. Add broth and red pepper flakes; increase heat and bring soup to a low boil.

Add cabbage and cook 2 minutes. Add shrimp, fish sauce, lime zest, and lime juice; cook just until shrimp turn pink, about 1 minute. Serve hot, sprinkled with cilantro, if using.

Makes 4 (2¼-cup) servings

NUTRITION AT A GLANCE

Per serving: 270 calories, 8 g fat, 1.5 g saturated fat, 38 g protein, 12 g carbohydrate, 1 g dietary fiber, 1,010 mg sodium

Asparagus Soup with Parmesan Sprinkle

PREP TIME: 10 minutes   **COOK TIME: 20 minutes**

Just a few simple ingredients create this rich and flavorful springtime soup. You can thin it with a little water if you prefer a thinner soup and use black pepper if you don't have white.

- 1 tablespoon extra-virgin olive oil
- 1 small onion, chopped
- 1 garlic clove, minced
- 2½ pounds asparagus, ends trimmed and cut into 1½-inch lengths
- 4 cups lower-sodium chicken broth
- 4 teaspoons freshly grated Parmesan cheese

  Salt and freshly ground white pepper

Heat oil over medium heat in a medium saucepan. Add onion, garlic, and asparagus and cook, stirring occasionally, until onions soften, 5 to 7 minutes. Do not brown.

Add broth, bring to a simmer, and cook until asparagus is just tender, about 10 minutes.

Remove from heat and carefully purée with a blender or hand blender. Return to the pan, gently reheat, and season with salt and pepper to taste. Serve each serving with a sprinkle of Parmesan.

Makes 4 (1¼-cup) servings

NUTRITION AT A GLANCE

Per serving: 90 calories, 2 g fat, 1 g saturated fat, 9 g protein, 12 g carbohydrate, 4 g dietary fiber, 170 mg sodium

Chicken and Mushroom Soup

PREP TIME: 10 minutes   **COOK TIME:** 20 minutes

Brussels sprouts add a rich background flavor and a hearty dose of vitamin A, fiber, folate, and other B vitamins to this basic soup. If you're unfamiliar with them or have never been a fan, give them a try in this recipe—you'll be amazed at how buttery and sweet they taste. Alternatively, omit the brussels sprouts and substitute an extra 2 cups of mushrooms.

1 medium leek, light green and white parts only, outer layer removed

4 cups lower-sodium chicken broth

1 cup water

½ teaspoon dried thyme

6 ounces white mushrooms, sliced

1 pound boneless, skinless chicken breasts, cut into ½-inch pieces

8 ounces brussels sprouts, halved

Salt and freshly ground black pepper

Trim leek, keeping root intact. Slice in half lengthwise, submerge in cold water, and rinse thoroughly to remove any dirt. Slice into ¼-inch pieces.

Bring broth, water, and thyme to a low boil in a large saucepan. Add leek and mushrooms; reduce heat and simmer until leek is softened, about 5 minutes. Add chicken and brussels sprouts. Simmer until chicken is cooked through, about 6 minutes. Season with salt and pepper to taste and serve hot.

Makes 4 (1¾-cup) servings

NUTRITION AT A GLANCE

Per serving: 210 calories, 3 g fat, 1 g saturated fat, 34 g protein, 13 g carbohydrate, 3 g dietary fiber, 240 mg sodium

Creamy Cauliflower Soup

PREP TIME: 5 minutes   **COOK TIME:** 30 minutes

Nutmeg and sautéed onions bring out the buttery, delicate flavor of cauliflower in this thick and satisfying soup.

1 (2-pound) head cauliflower

1 tablespoon extra-virgin olive oil

1 small onion, thinly sliced

¼ teaspoon salt

4 cups water

¼ cup reduced-fat sour cream

¼ teaspoon ground nutmeg

Salt and freshly ground black pepper

Cut cauliflower into florets and slice stems into ¼-inch pieces. Heat oil in a heavy-bottomed saucepan over medium heat. Add onion and cook until softened, stirring occasionally, about 5 minutes. Add cauliflower and ½ teaspoon salt; cover and cook for 5 minutes. Add water, cover, bring to a simmer, and cook until cauliflower is tender, about 15 minutes.

Purée vegetables and cooking liquid in a blender or food processor until smooth, or use a hand blender. Return to saucepan and whisk in sour cream and nutmeg. Season with salt and pepper to taste and serve.

Makes 4 (1¾-cup) servings

NUTRITION AT A GLANCE

Per serving: 110 calories, 6 g fat, 1.5 g saturated fat, 5 g protein, 14 g carbohydrate, 6 g dietary fiber, 290 mg sodium

Mexican Chicken Soup

PREP TIME: 10 minutes   **COOK TIME:** 15 minutes

Some soups make a meal, and this one certainly qualifies! Substitute shrimp for the chicken when you want to try something different; just add the shrimp when you add the salsa and simmer for 1 minute. Cilantro lovers can chop up some of the fresh herb and use it for sprinkling if desired.

- 1 tablespoon canola oil
- 1 small onion, chopped
- 1 jalapeño pepper, diced
- 2 garlic cloves, minced
- 2 teaspoons ground cumin
- 5 cups lower-sodium chicken broth
- 1½ pounds boneless, skinless chicken breasts, cut into 2-inch strips
- 2 cups mild refrigerated fresh salsa
- Salt and freshly ground black pepper

Heat oil in a large saucepan over medium heat. Add onion and jalapeño; cook, stirring often, until vegetables are tender, 5 minutes. Stir in garlic and cumin; cook 30 seconds more.

Add broth, increase heat to high, and bring to a rapid

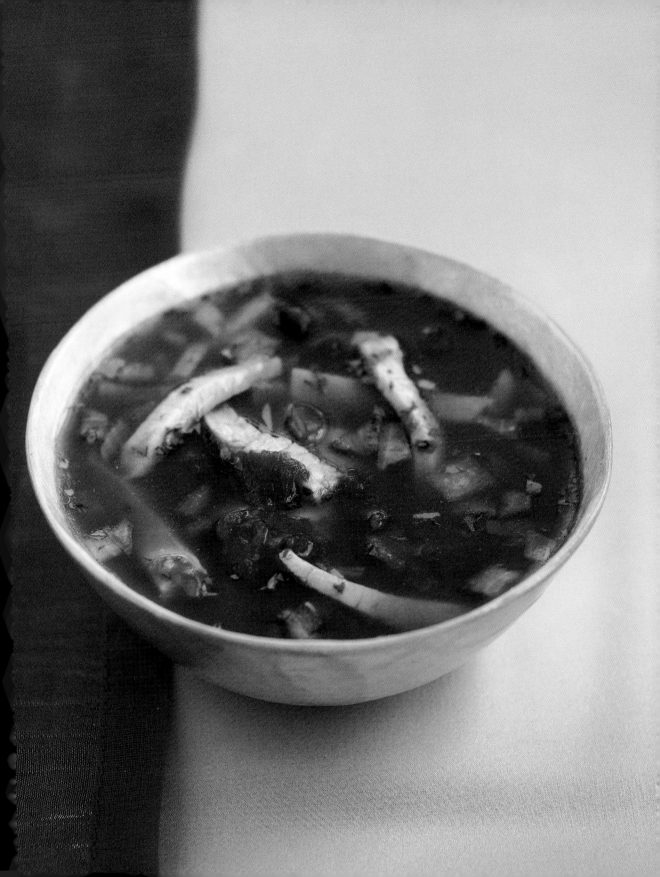

simmer. Add chicken and cook until no longer pink, about 3 minutes. Stir in salsa, bring back to a simmer, season with salt and pepper to taste, and serve hot.

Makes 4 (2¼-cup) servings

NUTRITION AT A GLANCE

Per serving: 320 calories, 8 g fat, 1.5 g saturated fat, 46 g protein, 14 g carbohydrate, 2 g dietary fiber, 680 mg sodium

Autumn Veggie Soup

PREP TIME: 10 minutes   **COOK TIME:** 20 minutes

Sweet potatoes, spinach, and edamame (fresh soybeans) make a tasty combination in this soup.

- 1 tablespoon extra-virgin olive oil
- 1 small onion, chopped
- 1 garlic clove, minced
- 4 cups vegetable broth
- 1 small sweet potato, peeled and cut into ½-inch cubes
- 1 cup frozen shelled edamame beans
- 2 ounces baby spinach (2 cups)
- Salt and freshly ground black pepper

Heat oil in a medium saucepan over medium heat. Add onion and garlic, reduce heat to medium-low, and cook, stirring frequently, until softened, about 5 minutes. Do not brown.

Add broth, increase heat to high, and bring to boil. Add sweet potato and edamame, reduce to a simmer, and cook until vegetables are tender, about 5 minutes. Stir in spinach and heat until wilted.

Season with salt and pepper to taste and serve.

Makes 4 (1½-cup) servings

NUTRITION AT A GLANCE

Per serving: 150 calories, 7 g fat, 1 g saturated fat, 6 g protein, 17 g carbohydrate, 3 g dietary fiber, 560 mg sodium

Rustic Tomato Soup

PREP TIME: 5 minutes   **COOK TIME:** 20 minutes

For a creamy version of this simple Italian-style soup, stir 1 tablespoon of plain low-fat yogurt and ½ teaspoon of granular sugar substitute into each bowl before serving.

> 1 tablespoon extra-virgin olive oil
>
> 3 garlic cloves, coarsely chopped
>
> ¼ teaspoon red pepper flakes (optional)
>
> 1 (28-ounce) can unsalted diced tomatoes
>
> 2 tablespoons chopped fresh basil
>
> 2 (5.5-ounce) cans low-sodium vegetable juice
>
> Salt and freshly ground black pepper

Heat oil in a medium saucepan over medium-low heat. Add garlic and red pepper flakes, if using; stir occasionally until softened, about 3 minutes. Add tomatoes with juice, basil, and vegetable juice. Increase heat to medium and simmer for 15 minutes. Season with salt and pepper to taste and serve hot.

Makes 4 (1-cup) servings

NUTRITION AT A GLANCE

Per serving: 90 calories, 3.5 g fat, .5 g saturated fat, 2 g protein, 14 g carbohydrate, 4 g dietary fiber, 210 mg sodium

Apple–Butternut Squash Soup

PREP TIME: 10 minutes   **COOK TIME:** 35 minutes

Unsweetened apple cider adds body and a natural hint of sweetness to this thick and flavorful soup, and creamy winter squash delivers ample amounts of beta-carotene, B vitamins, and fiber. This recipe is very easy but it does take slightly longer to cook, which allows the flavors to meld perfectly. Look for packaged cut squash to help you save prep time.

1 tablespoon extra-virgin olive oil

1 small onion, thinly sliced

2 pounds butternut squash, peeled, seeded, and cut into 1-inch pieces

3 cups lower-sodium chicken broth

½ cup unsweetened apple cider

Salt and freshly ground black pepper

Heat oil in a large heavy-bottomed saucepan over medium heat. Add onion and cook until softened and lightly browned, about 5 minutes. Add squash, cover, and cook 10 minutes more, stirring occasionally. Add broth and simmer until softened, 15 to 20 minutes.

Using a slotted spoon, transfer solid ingredients to a blender with apple cider and purée until smooth. Add

1⅓ cups of the cooking liquid and purée until smooth. Stir back into the pan. Serve hot.

Makes 6 (1½-cup) servings

NUTRITION AT A GLANCE

Per serving: 160 calories, 5 g fat, 1 g saturated fat, 6 g protein, 28 g carbohydrate, 4 g dietary fiber, 135 mg sodium

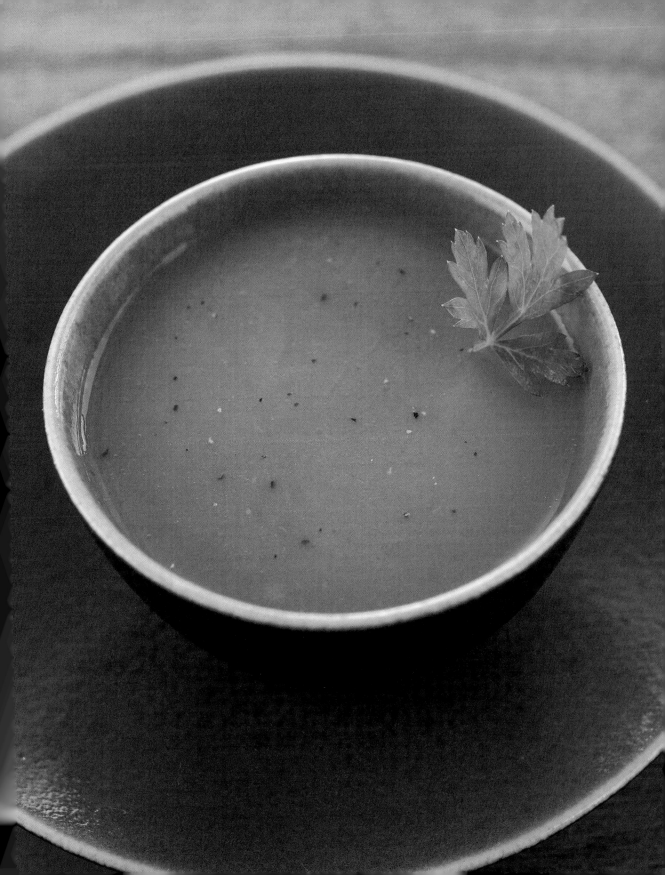

Chilled Cucumber and Mint Soup

PREP TIME: 25 minutes

When things heat up in Miami, we turn to this tasty combination of refreshing cucumbers, aromatic mint, and tangy reduced-fat sour cream. It makes a "cool" companion to a lunchtime sandwich or salad. Or try it as a prelude to anything barbecued on a sultry summer night.

- 3 cucumbers, peeled, seeded, and roughly chopped
- 1 scallion, sliced
- 1 garlic clove, chopped
- 3 tablespoons fresh mint leaves
- ½ cup water
- 1 (8-ounce) container reduced-fat sour cream
- 1 tablespoon fresh lemon juice
- ¼ teaspoon salt
- ¼ teaspoon freshly ground white pepper

Purée cucumbers, scallion, garlic, mint, and water in a blender or food processor until smooth. Add sour cream, lemon juice, salt, and pepper and blend to combine.

If you are serving the soup immediately, chill quickly by transferring soup to a metal mixing bowl, placing bowl over a larger bowl filled with ice and cold water, and stirring occasionally until chilled, about 10 minutes. Otherwise, chill in refrigerator until cold, about 3 hours.

Makes 4 (1-cup) servings

NUTRITION AT A GLANCE

Per serving: 100 calories, 7 g fat, 4.5 g saturated fat, 3 g protein, 8 g carbohydrate, 2 g dietary fiber, 180 mg sodium

Curried Zucchini Soup

PREP TIME: 10 minutes   **COOK TIME: 20 minutes**

Zucchini takes on Indian flavors exceptionally well, and there is almost no better example than this fantastic curried soup. Garam masala is an Indian spice blend that's widely available at specialty food stores, but if you don't have it, the soup is still great.

- 2 teaspoons extra-virgin olive oil
- 1 small onion, chopped
- 1 garlic clove, minced
- 2 medium zucchini, sliced into ¼-inch half-moons
- 1 tablespoon grated fresh ginger
- 1 teaspoon curry powder
- ½ teaspoon garam masala (optional)
- 3 cups vegetable broth
- ½ cup plain fat-free or low-fat yogurt

Heat oil in a large saucepan over medium heat. Add onion and garlic; cook until softened, about 5 minutes. Add zucchini, ginger, curry powder, and garam masala, if using. Cook 3 more minutes.

Add broth and bring to a simmer. Cover and simmer until vegetables are tender, about 10 minutes. Purée soup in a blender or food processor until smooth, or use a hand blender. Whisk in yogurt just before serving.

Makes 4 (generous 1¼-cup) servings

NUTRITION AT A GLANCE

Per serving: 90 calories, 2.5 g fat, 0 g saturated fat, 3 g protein, 12 g carbohydrate, 2 g dietary fiber, 540 mg sodium

Shrimp Gazpacho

PREP TIME: 5 minutes   **COOK TIME:** 5 minutes

If you don't believe you can open your pantry and mix together a few basics to make a delicious, refreshing soup, then try this recipe! Adding shrimp transforms this chilled classic into a meal. Make it a day in advance if you'd like, but keep the shrimp separate until just before serving.

- 16 large peeled and deveined fresh or thawed frozen shrimp
- 1 tablespoon plus 1 teaspoon extra-virgin olive oil, divided
- 3 cups low-sodium tomato or vegetable juice, chilled
- 1 medium cucumber, peeled, seeded, and chopped
- ¾ cup medium salsa
- ¼ cup ice water
- 1 tablespoon red wine vinegar

  Salt and freshly ground black pepper

Toss shrimp with 1 teaspoon of the oil and season with salt and pepper. Heat a nonstick skillet or grill pan over medium-high heat. Add shrimp and cook for 1 minute per side. Remove to a plate to cool.

Combine remaining oil, tomato juice, cucumber, salsa, water, and vinegar in a large mixing bowl; season with salt and pepper to taste. Divide among bowls, top with shrimp, and serve.

Makes 4 (2 cup) servings

NUTRITION AT A GLANCE

Per serving: 130 calories, 5 g fat, ½ g saturated fat, 8 g protein, 14 g carbohydrate, 3 g dietary fiber, 460 mg sodium

Vegetable and Bean Soup

PREP TIME: 5 minutes   **COOK TIME: 25 minutes**

This satisfying vegetarian soup is filled with hearty beans and vegetables. The stems of Swiss chard are tender and filled with nutrients, so cut just the thick ends off and thinly slice the rest before chopping the leaves. Adding the chard at the end lends a bright note of fresh flavor.

1 (1-pound) bunch Swiss chard, thick stem ends removed and discarded

2 teaspoons extra-virgin olive oil, plus extra for drizzling

2 celery stalks, chopped

1 small onion, chopped

1 garlic clove, minced

3 cups low-sodium tomato vegetable juice

1 (14½-ounce) can unsalted diced tomatoes

1 (15-ounce) can navy or other small white beans, rinsed and drained

½ teaspoon dried oregano

Salt and freshly ground black pepper

Submerge chard in cold water and rinse thoroughly; thinly slice stems and coarsely chop leaves.

Heat 2 teaspoons of the oil in a large saucepan over medium-high heat. Add celery and onion and cook, stirring often, until softened, about 5 minutes. Add garlic and cook 1 minute more. Add broth, tomatoes with juice, beans, and oregano; bring to a low boil.

Reduce heat to medium-low, cover, and simmer for 10 minutes. Add chard and cook 5 minutes more. Season with salt and pepper, drizzle with oil, and serve hot.

Makes 4 (1¾-cup) servings

NUTRITION AT A GLANCE

Per serving: 200 calories, 3.5 g fat, 0 g saturated fat, 10 g protein, 31 g carbohydrate, 8 g dietary fiber, 820 mg sodium

Cilantro Pesto Dip

PREP TIME: 5 minutes   **COOK TIME:** 15 minutes

This zesty, versatile dip is great with crudités as a snack or for a party. You can also dollop it on grilled fish or chicken or toss it with cubed cooked chicken for an easy and unique chicken salad. In later phases, use it as a sandwich spread or as a chili or burrito topping. It keeps 5 days in the refrigerator and freezes for up to a month.

⅓ cup walnuts

1 large bunch cilantro, leaves and stems intact

1 garlic clove, peeled

¼ cup extra-virgin olive oil

3 tablespoons reduced-fat sour cream

2 teaspoons fresh lemon juice

¼ teaspoon salt

Heat oven or toaster oven to 275°F. Spread walnuts on a baking tray and bake until fragrant and lightly browned, about 10 minutes. Cool slightly, about 3 minutes.

Chop cilantro, garlic, and walnuts in a food processor, about 25 seconds. With machine running, add oil in a

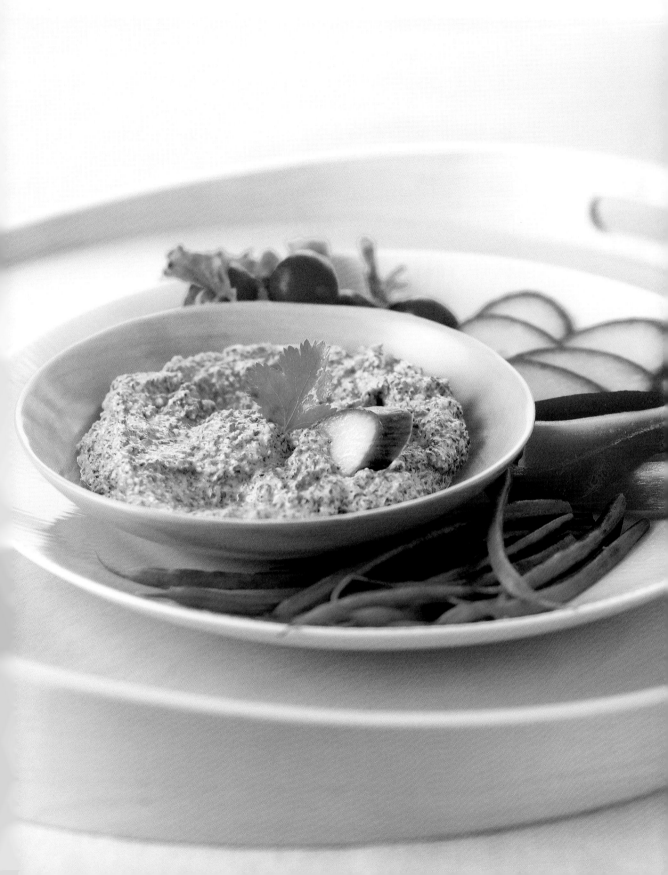

steady stream. Add sour cream, lemon juice, and salt. Pulse a few times to combine. Serve or refrigerate until needed.

Makes 8 (2½-tablespoon) servings

NUTRITION AT A GLANCE

Per serving: 100 calories, 10 g fat, 1.5 g saturated fat, 1 g protein, 1 g carbohydrate, 0 g dietary, 80 mg sodium

Green Apple and Peanut Butter Sandwich

PREP TIME: 5 minutes

This tasty open-faced "sandwich" is a quick and easy pick-me-up snack when midday hunger strikes and time is tight. Note: Count the 1 tablespoon of peanut butter as half of your total nuts allowed for the day.

- 1 tablespoon creamy or crunchy trans-fat-free peanut butter
- 1 large whole-grain crispbread cracker
- ⅛ Granny Smith apple, thinly sliced

Spread peanut butter on cracker and top with apple slices.

Makes 1 serving

NUTRITION AT A GLANCE

Per serving: 130 calories, 8 g fat, 1 g saturated fat, 5 g protein, 13 g carbohydrate, 3 g dietary fiber, 65 mg sodium

Pecan-Stuffed Dates

PREP TIME: 5 minutes   **COOK TIME: 20 minutes**

This sweet and crunchy snack couldn't be simpler. Nutritionally, dates offer potassium and fiber, and pecans provide heart-healthy monounsaturated and polyunsaturated fats, which can lower blood cholesterol.

24 pecan halves

24 dates, pitted

Heat oven or toaster oven to 350°F. Spread pecans on a baking tray and bake until lightly toasted and fragrant, about 10 minutes. Cool 5 minutes.

Slice dates lengthwise but not all the way through. Place 1 pecan inside each date and use your fingers to close and reseal dates. Store in an airtight container at room temperature for up to 2 weeks.

Makes 8 (3-piece) servings

NUTRITION AT A GLANCE

Per serving: 160 calories, 3 g fat, 0 g saturated fat, 1 g protein, 35 g carbohydrate, 4 g dietary fiber, 0 mg sodium

Celery with Herbed Cream Cheese and Walnuts

PREP TIME: 5 minutes   **COOK TIME: 15 minutes**

This tasty grown-up version of an old-time favorite is great for a party or a take-along snack. You can try the cream cheese mixture as a spread on whole-grain crackers or use it for tea sandwiches on whole-grain bread.

⅓ cup walnuts

1 (8-ounce) package reduced-fat cream cheese, at room temperature

1 tablespoon chopped fresh chives

16 large celery stalks, trimmed

Salt and freshly ground black pepper

Heat oven or toaster oven to 275°F. Spread walnuts on a baking tray and bake until fragrant and toasted, about 10 minutes. Roughly chop.

Combine walnuts, cream cheese, and chives in a mixing bowl. Mix well. Add salt and pepper to taste.

Using a rubber spatula, fill each celery stalk with 1 tablespoon cream cheese mixture and serve.

Makes 8 servings

NUTRITION AT A GLANCE

Per serving: 90 calories, 6 g fat, 2 g saturated fat, 5 g protein, 6 g carbohydrate, 2 g dietary fiber, 240 mg sodium

Soy Chai Tea, Two Ways

Spiced with ginger, cinnamon, cardamom, cloves, and black pepper, our soy chai teas—both hot and iced—make a healthy, energy-boosting snack on a cold winter or sultry summer day. Keep extra iced soy tea in the refrigerator for up to 1 week.

Hot Soy Chai

PREP TIME: 10 minutes

- 1 cup low-fat, low-sugar plain soymilk
- 1 decaffeinated chai tea bag
- ¼ teaspoon granular sugar substitute (optional)

Heat soymilk until just boiling. Pour over tea bag, cover, and steep 5 minutes. Gently squeeze tea bag, remove, and discard. Serve tea hot with sugar substitute, if desired.

Makes 1 (1-cup) serving

NUTRITION AT A GLANCE

Per serving: 100 calories, 1.5 g fat, 0 g saturated fat, 7 g protein, 16 g carbohydrate, 2 g dietary fiber, 80 mg sodium

Iced Soy Chai

PREP TIME: 15 minutes

- 32 ounces (4 cups) low-fat, low-sugar plain soymilk
- 6 decaffeinated chai tea bags
- 1 teaspoon granular sugar substitute (optional)

Heat soymilk until just boiling. Add tea bags, cover, and steep 5 minutes. Gently squeeze tea bags, remove, and discard. Stir in sugar substitute, if using, and serve over ice.

Makes 4 (1-cup) servings

NUTRITION AT A GLANCE

Per serving: 100 calories, 1.5 g fat, 0 g saturated fat, 7 g protein, 16 g carbohydrate, 2 g dietary fiber, 80 mg sodium

Multigrain Watercress and Cucumber Tea Sandwiches

PREP TIME: 10 minutes

Tea sandwiches may sound like dainty little bites, but this version, which replaces butter with reduced-fat cream cheese and white bread with whole grain, makes a healthy and very tasty snack or lunch.

8 thin slices multigrain bread

4 ounces reduced-fat cream cheese, at room temperature

½ bunch watercress, tough stems removed

1 medium cucumber, thinly sliced

Spread each slice of bread with cream cheese; make sandwiches with watercress and cucumber. Remove crusts, if desired, and cut each sandwich into 3 rectangular slices.

Makes 4 lunch servings or 6 snack servings

NUTRITION AT A GLANCE

Per lunch serving: 170 calories, 6 g fat, 3.5 g saturated fat, 8 g protein, 25 g carbohydrate, 6 g dietary fiber, 20 mg cholesterol, 330 mg sodium

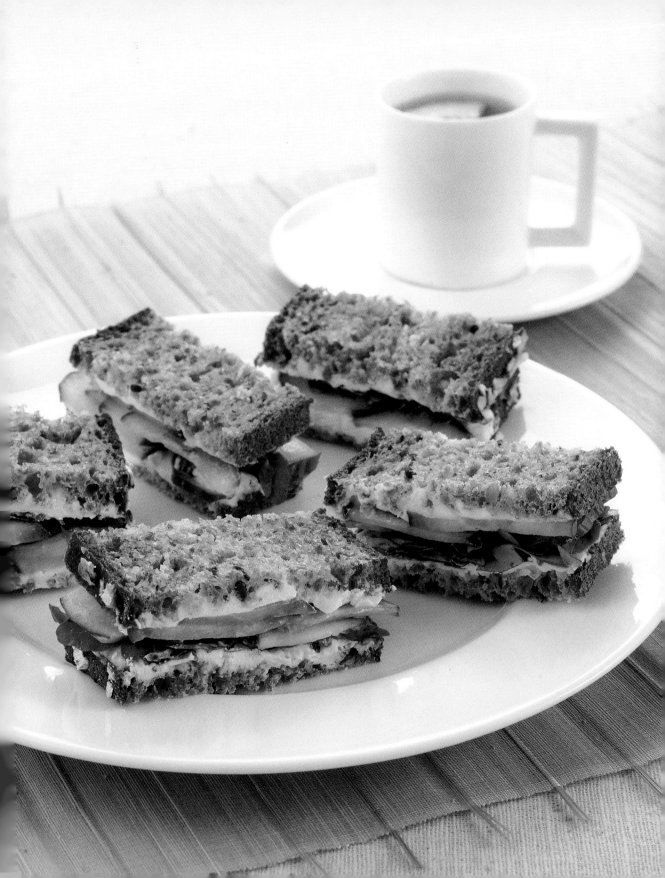

Peppery Cheese Popcorn

PREP TIME: 5 minutes   **COOK TIME: 5 minutes**

Everyone loves popcorn as a movie snack, especially when it's "doctored up," making it both fun and satisfying. Casablanca, anyone?

6	cups freshly air-popped popcorn (⅓ cup unpopped kernels)
	Butter-flavored cooking spray
2	tablespoons finely grated Parmesan cheese
¼	teaspoon freshly ground black pepper
	Salt

Place popcorn in a large mixing bowl and coat lightly with cooking spray. Sprinkle with cheese and pepper and toss to combine. Season with salt and more pepper to taste; serve.

Makes 2 (3-cup) servings

NUTRITION AT A GLANCE

Per serving: 120 calories, 3 g fat, 1 g saturated fat, 5 g protein, 19 g carbohydrate, 4 g dietary fiber, 220 mg sodium

Warm Artichoke Dip

PREP TIME: 10 minutes   COOK TIME: 5 minutes

This creamy South Beach version of a favorite classic dip is just as good as the real thing. Dress it up with a finishing touch of your own, such as a sprinkle of paprika, chopped parsley, or sliced scallions.

1 (8-ounce) package reduced-fat cream cheese

½ cup mayonnaise

½ cup 1 percent milk

1 ounce freshly grated Parmesan cheese (¼ cup)

1 garlic clove, minced

1 teaspoon hot pepper sauce

1 (14-ounce) can artichoke hearts, drained

1 teaspoon fresh lemon juice

Salt and freshly ground black pepper

Assorted whole-grain crackers

Blend cream cheese, mayonnaise, milk, cheese, garlic, and hot pepper sauce in a food processor until smooth. Add artichokes and pulse until well combined but still chunky.

Transfer to a microwave-safe serving dish. Microwave on medium heat until heated through, turning once or twice, about 5 minutes. Stir in lemon juice and season to taste with salt and pepper. Serve with crackers.

Makes 12 (¼-cup) servings

NUTRITION AT A GLANCE

Per serving: 140 calories, 11 g fat, 3.5 g saturated fat, 4 g protein, 5 g carbohydrate, 0 g dietary fiber, 350 mg sodium

Southwest Pepita and Pecan Mix

PREP TIME: 5 minutes   **COOK TIME: 20 minutes**

The sweet and smoky aromas of the Southwest will fill your kitchen as you bake this zesty snack. Make it for a party or pack it into individual snack bags and take it to work. Nutrient-rich pumpkin seeds provide fiber, protein, minerals, omega-3 fatty acids, and more.

- 1 tablespoon chili powder
- 2 teaspoons salt
- 2 teaspoons ground cumin
- ⅛ teaspoon cayenne pepper
- 1 large egg white
- 2 cups shelled, unsalted raw pumpkin seeds
- 1½ cups pecan halves
- 1 cup shelled, unsalted sunflower seeds

Position rack in center of oven and heat to 375°F. Lightly coat a baking sheet with cooking spray or vegetable oil. Combine chili powder, salt, cumin, and cayenne in a mixing bowl.

Whisk egg white in a large mixing bowl until foamy, about 15 seconds. Add pumpkin seeds, pecans, and sunflower seeds; mix with a slotted spoon to combine. Sprinkle one-third of the spice mixture over seed mixture and toss to combine and coat evenly. Repeat with remaining spice mixture.

Spread seed mixture on the baking sheet in a single layer. Bake for 10 minutes, break up into clumps, turn pan, and continue baking until seed mixture is crisp and browned, about 10 minutes more.

Remove from oven and cool. Break up into pieces with your fingers and serve. This snack mix can be stored in an airtight container for up to 2 weeks at room temperature or 1 month in the freezer. Heat in a 375°F oven for 5 minutes to recrisp, if necessary.

Makes 20 (¼-cup) servings

NUTRITION AT A GLANCE

Per serving: 170 calories, 16 g fat, 2 g saturated fat, 6 g protein, 5 g carbohydrate, 2 g dietary fiber, 240 mg sodium

Creamy Tex-Mex Bean Dip with Baked Tortilla Chips

PREP TIME: 5 minutes   **COOK TIME:** 12 minutes

When you need to make a quick appetizer with simple pantry staples, this dip is the answer. Hot salsa gives it just the right kick, and cream cheese makes it rich and creamy. Black soybeans bump up the protein, but you can also use regular black beans, if you wish.

- 4 (8-inch) whole-wheat tortillas, cut into 8 wedges each
- 1 (15-ounce) can black soybeans, rinsed and drained
- 4 ounces reduced-fat cream cheese, cut into cubes
- ½ cup hot salsa
- 1 tablespoon fresh lime juice
- 1 teaspoon ground cumin
- ½ teaspoon chili powder
- 2 tablespoons shredded reduced-fat cheddar cheese

Heat oven to 350°F. Arrange tortilla wedges on a baking sheet and bake until crisp, about 12 minutes.

While chips are baking, blend together beans, cream cheese, salsa, lime juice, cumin, and chili powder in a food processor until smooth. Transfer mixture to a nonstick skillet and heat over medium-low heat, stirring constantly, until hot, 5 minutes (do not boil).

Transfer dip to a serving dish, sprinkle with cheese, and serve hot with tortilla chips.

Makes 8 (¼-cup) servings of dip

NUTRITION AT A GLANCE

Per serving: 140 calories, 5 g fat, 2 g saturated fat, 7 g protein, 16 g carbohydrate, 3 g dietary fiber, 220 mg sodium

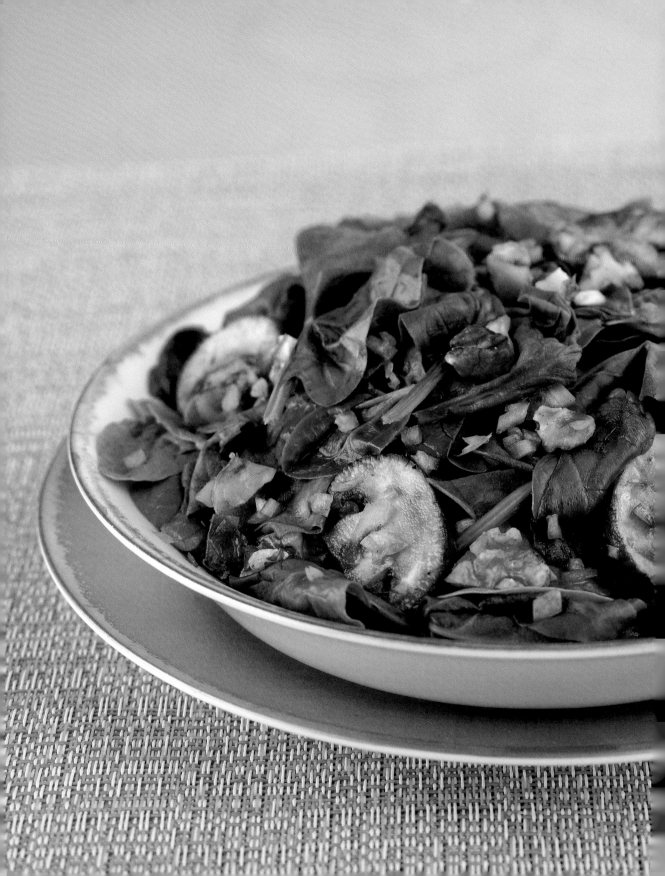

SALADS

From old-time favorites to new inspirations, there's never a dull moment when it comes to the salads in the pages ahead. Some of them make a complete lunch or light dinner; others might inspire a theme for the rest of your meal.

We've included classics, like our Phase 1 Caesar salad; vitamin-packed recipes, such as spinach tossed with tender grilled chicken and juicy pomegranate seeds; and fresh veggies in unique combinations, like tender red leaf lettuce, creamy avocado, and crisp apple.

When you want to make salad a meal, go for high-protein options: Chicken Tahini or Tuna Pasta Salads, for example. Those that can stand in as sides when served in smaller portions include Moroccan Cabbage and Carrot Slaw and Jicama, Tomato, and Black Bean Salad.

◀ *Warm Spinach Salad with Mushrooms (page 154)*

Warm Spinach Salad with Mushrooms

PREP TIME: 5 minutes   **COOK TIME:** 10 minutes

Walnuts add crunch and a buttery taste to this spinach lovers' favorite. Serve it alongside grilled steak or add a sliced chicken breast and you've got a tasty meal. Use whole leaf spinach, if you'd like; just stem and tear into bite-size pieces before proceeding.

> 1 shallot, minced
>
> 1 teaspoon red wine vinegar
>
> 12 ounces baby spinach (10 to 12 cups)
>
> 2 tablespoons extra-virgin olive oil, divided
>
> ¼ cup walnuts, roughly chopped
>
> 8 ounces white mushrooms, sliced
>
> Salt and freshly ground black pepper

Combine shallot, vinegar, and ¼ teaspoon salt in a small bowl. Place spinach in a large mixing bowl.

Heat 1 tablespoon of the oil in a large skillet over medium heat. Add walnuts and cook, stirring frequently, until lightly browned, about 3 minutes. Remove from the pan with a slotted spoon and add to spinach.

Add mushrooms to the skillet and cook over medium heat until softened and lightly browned, 3 to 5 minutes. Transfer mushrooms and warm oil to bowl with spinach, making sure to use all of the oil. Add shallot mixture and remaining oil; gently toss to combine. Season with salt and pepper to taste and serve immediately.

Makes 4 (2-cup) servings

NUTRITION AT A GLANCE

Per serving: 160 calories, 12 g fat, 1.5 g saturated fat, 4 g protein, 13 g carbohydrate, 5 g dietary fiber, 210 mg sodium

Jicama, Tomato, and Black Bean Salad

PREP TIME: 15 minutes

Jicama, a delightfully crunchy Mexican root vegetable, is often eaten raw in salads and slaws. Tossed with a zesty lime dressing and mixed with beans and juicy tomatoes, it makes an easy, irresistible salad that's perfect with anything from the grill. Prepare a double batch and take it along to your next potluck—just be ready to share the recipe!

3 tablespoons fresh lime juice

1 garlic clove, minced

½ teaspoon ground cumin

3 tablespoons extra-virgin olive oil

1 (15-ounce) can black beans, rinsed and drained

1 small jicama, peeled and chopped

2 plum tomatoes, chopped

3 tablespoons diced red onion

¼ cup chopped fresh cilantro

Salt and freshly ground black pepper

Whisk together lime juice, garlic, and cumin in a large mixing bowl; slowly whisk in oil. Add beans, jicama,

tomatoes, onion, and cilantro. Toss to combine, season
with salt and pepper, and serve.

Makes 4 (1-cup) servings

NUTRITION AT A GLANCE

Per serving: 190 calories, 11 g fat, 1.5 g saturated fat,
4 g protein, 22 g carbohydrate, 9 g dietary fiber,
400 mg sodium

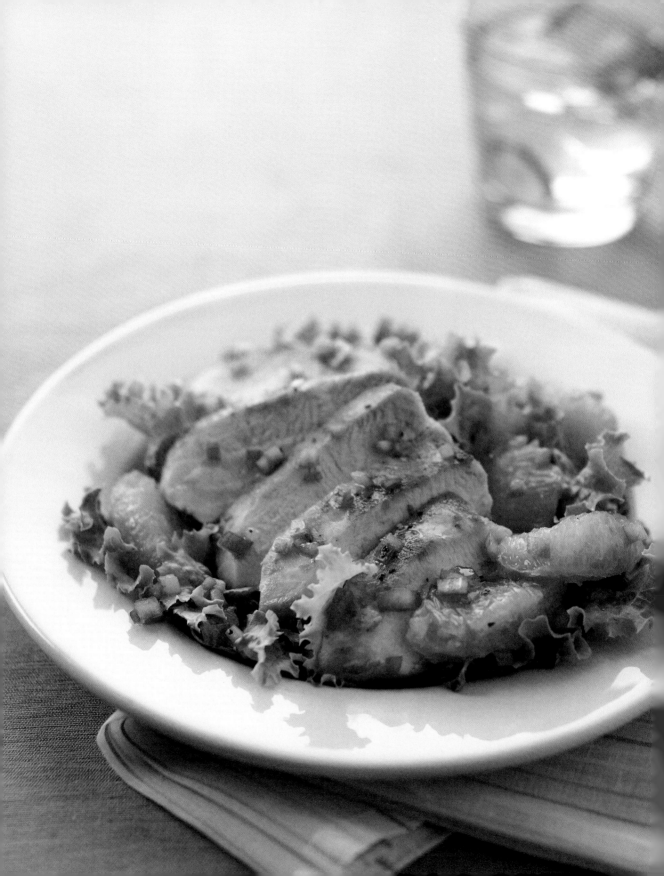

Greens, Chicken, and Citrus Salad

PREP TIME: 15 minutes   **COOK TIME:** 15 minutes

Grapefruit brings a refreshing taste, a pretty look, and a healthy dose of vitamin C and fiber to this salad. To easily section the grapefruit, use a paring knife to cut the peel from the flesh and trim excess pith. Placing the knife blade between fruit section and membrane, carefully cut each section out one by one. Using leftover cooked chicken breasts cuts the total time for this recipe in half.

- 2 tablespoons minced red onion
- 2 tablespoons sherry vinegar
- 5 tablespoons extra-virgin olive oil, divided
- 1½ pounds boneless, skinless chicken breasts
- 1 (1-pound) head green leaf lettuce, torn into bite-size pieces (8 cups)
- 1 pink grapefruit, sectioned

  Salt and freshly ground black pepper

Combine onion, vinegar, 4 tablespoons of the oil, ¼ teaspoon salt, and ⅛ teaspoon pepper in a jar with a lid. Close tightly and shake vigorously to combine.

Season chicken with salt and pepper. Heat remaining oil in a large skillet over medium-high heat; cook chicken until browned, 5 to 7 minutes per side. Remove from heat, cut into ½-inch slices, and toss with 3 tablespoons of the dressing.

Gently toss together lettuce, grapefruit, and remaining dressing in a large bowl. Season to taste with salt and pepper. Serve salad topped with chicken slices.

Makes 4 (2-cup) servings

NUTRITION AT A GLANCE

Per serving: 380 calories, 20 g fat, 3 g saturated fat, 41 g protein, 8 g carbohydrate, 2 g dietary fiber, 190 mg sodium

Eggless Caesar Salad

PREP TIME: 15 minutes

You won't miss the eggs in this creamy Caesar salad. Top it with grilled chicken or shrimp to make a hearty lunch or light dinner. In later phases, you can add a quick multigrain crouton: Just cut 2 slices multigrain bread into ½-inch cubes, toss with 1 tablespoon extra-virgin olive oil, and toast in a 400°F oven until crisp, about 8 minutes.

- 1 tablespoon fresh lemon juice
- 2 anchovy fillets, minced
- 1 garlic clove, minced
- ½ teaspoon Dijon mustard
- ¼ cup extra-virgin olive oil
- 1 tablespoon freshly grated Parmesan cheese
- 1 (1½-pound) head romaine lettuce, chopped (8 to 10 cups)
- Salt and freshly ground black pepper

Whisk together lemon juice, anchovy, garlic, and mustard in a large mixing bowl; slowly whisk in oil. Stir

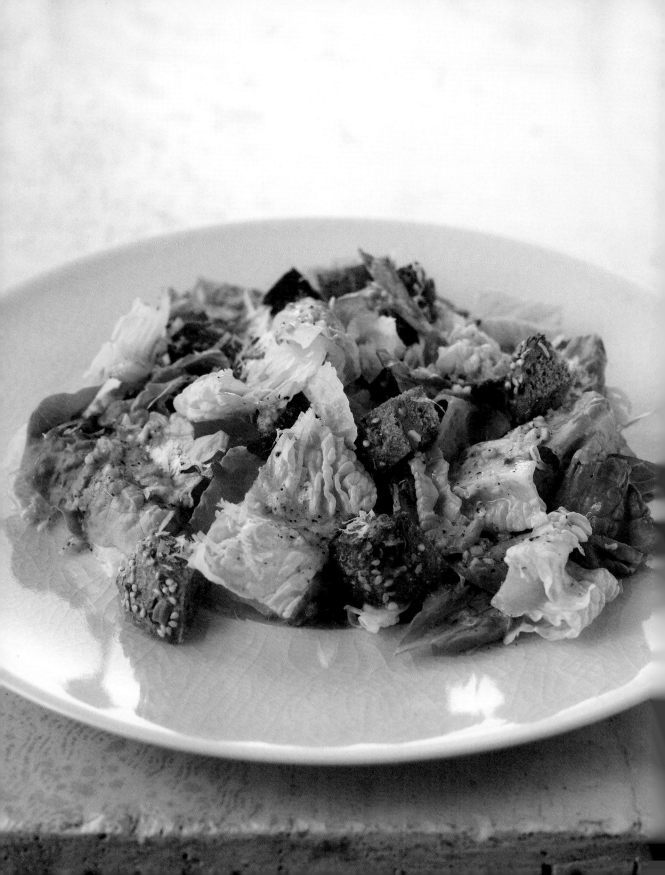

in cheese and season to taste with salt and pepper. Add lettuce, toss, and serve.

Makes 4 (2-cup) servings

NUTRITION AT A GLANCE

Per serving: 160 calories, 15 g fat, 2.5 g saturated fat, 3 g protein, 4 g carbohydrate, 2 g dietary fiber, 125 mg sodium

Ribbon Salad

PREP TIME: 15 minutes

Slicing lettuce leaves into thin ribbons gives this simple salad a fresh, lively look, and its lemony dressing lends a vibrant taste. Use this simple recipe as a base, adding fresh herbs, toasted nuts, cherry tomatoes, or chopped cucumber when you want a change of pace.

  1 (¾-pound) head red leaf lettuce (6 cups)

  2 tablespoons extra-virgin olive oil

  1 tablespoon fresh lemon juice

     Salt and freshly ground black pepper

Core lettuce and break apart into whole leaves. Wash and dry leaves, then pile half of them in an even layered pile. Slice leaves crosswise into ¼-inch strips. Repeat with remaining leaves.

  Place lettuce strips in a large mixing bowl and add oil and lemon juice; toss to combine. Season with salt and pepper and serve.

Makes 4 (2-cup) servings

NUTRITION AT A GLANCE

Per serving: 70 calories, 7 g fat, 1 g saturated fat, 0 g protein, 0 g carbohydrate, 0 g dietary fiber, 75 mg sodium

Tuna Pasta Salad

PREP TIME: 15 minutes   **COOK TIME:** 15 minutes

Not your average pasta or tuna salad, this combination is filled with crunchy celery, juicy tomatoes, and fresh sweet peas. Flavorful and filling, it's perfect for the office or a picnic lunch. If you're making pasta for dinner, make some extra to use in this salad the next day, and your total time will only be about 15 minutes.

- 8 ounces spelt or whole-wheat pasta
- ¼ cup mayonnaise
- ¼ cup plain fat-free or low-fat yogurt
- 1 tablespoon plus 1 teaspoon balsamic vinegar
- 2 (6-ounce) cans solid white tuna packed in water, drained
- 4 large celery stalks, chopped
- 6 ounces cherry tomatoes (about 15 tomatoes), quartered
- ⅔ cup frozen peas, thawed
- 2 tablespoons minced red onion

  Salt and freshly ground black pepper

Cook pasta according to package directions until tender but still firm to the bite. Drain and rinse under cold water for 30 seconds.

Whisk together mayonnaise, yogurt, and vinegar in a small mixing bowl. Season to taste with salt and pepper.

Place tuna in a large mixing bowl and break into

small pieces. Add pasta, celery, tomatoes, peas, and onion; stir to combine. Add dressing and stir to combine. Season to taste with salt and pepper and refrigerate until ready to serve.

Makes 4 (1¾-cup) servings

NUTRITION AT A GLANCE

Per serving: 450 calories, 15 g fat, 2 g saturated fat, 31 g protein, 50 g carbohydrate, 7 g dietary fiber, 570 mg sodium

Bulgur, Cucumber, and Mint Salad

PREP TIME: 10 minutes   **COOK TIME:** 25 minutes

A great "take along" to the office or the beach, this fresh lemony salad also works well as a delicious side dish. Try it with Halibut with Tapenade in Parchment (page 214) or Yogurt-Marinated Lamb Kebabs (page 324). For best flavor, look for ripe tomatoes in season.

1½ cups water

¾ cup bulgur wheat

1 medium tomato, cut into ½-inch cubes

1 medium cucumber, peeled, seeded, and cut into ½-inch cubes

2 tablespoons chopped fresh mint

2 tablespoons extra-virgin olive oil

1 tablespoon fresh lemon juice

Salt and freshly ground black pepper

Bring water and bulgur to a boil in a medium saucepan, reduce heat to low, cover, and simmer until bulgur is cooked and water is absorbed, about 12 minutes. Remove from heat.

Spread bulgur onto a large plate and place in refrigerator to cool slightly, about 5 minutes. Place in a mixing bowl and fluff with a fork. Add tomato, cucumber, mint, oil, and lemon juice; stir together and season with salt and pepper to taste. Serve at room temperature.

Makes 4 (1-cup) servings

NUTRITION AT A GLANCE

Per serving: 160 calories, 7 g fat, 1 g saturated fat, 4 g protein, 22 g carbohydrate, 5 g dietary fiber, 80 mg sodium

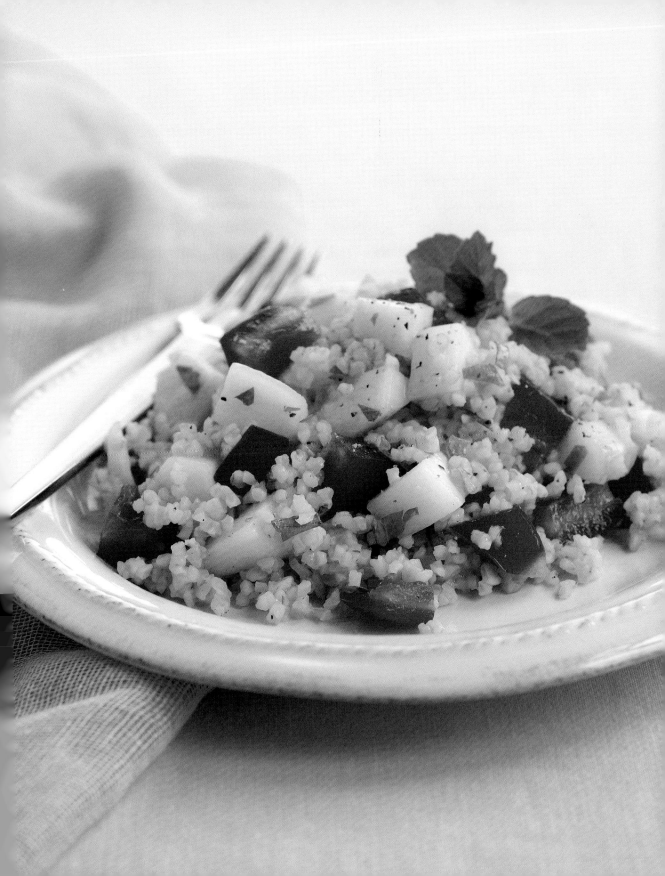

Crispy Tempeh Salad

PREP TIME: 15 minutes   **COOK TIME:** 10 minutes

Combine nutty tempeh, crisp cucumber, and a lemony Dijon dressing and you end up with a hearty, protein-packed main dish that will make even nonvegetarians swoon. For extra flavor, marinate the tempeh for up to an hour if you have time.

2 tablespoons extra-virgin olive oil, divided

1 tablespoon fresh lemon juice

1 teaspoon Dijon mustard

½ (8-ounce) package soy tempeh

5 ounces mesclun/mixed salad greens (5 to 6 cups)

1 small cucumber, peeled, seeded, and sliced

Salt and freshly ground black pepper

Place 1½ tablespoons oil, lemon juice, mustard, ¼ teaspoon salt, and a pinch of pepper in a small jar. Close tightly and shake vigorously to combine.

Place tempeh in a shallow dish and add 1 tablespoon of the dressing; season both sides with salt and pepper and turn to coat. Marinate at room temperature for 10 minutes.

Heat remaining oil in a medium nonstick skillet over medium heat; add tempeh and cook until golden brown, about 4 minutes per side. Remove from pan and slice into 4 triangular pieces. Brush with ½ tablespoon of the dressing.

Place greens and cucumber in a mixing bowl. Add remaining dressing and toss to combine. Add salt and pepper to taste and serve with tempeh.

Makes 2 (2½-cup) servings

NUTRITION AT A GLANCE

Per serving: 260 calories, 20 g fat, 3 g saturated fat, 12 g protein, 11 g carbohydrate, 2 g dietary fiber, 240 mg sodium

Feta, Cucumber, and Radish Salad

PREP TIME: 15 minutes

Creamy feta cheese matches perfectly with crisp cucumber, peppery radish, and fresh-tasting mint in this refreshing salad. Try it with Lamb Chops with Chimichurri Sauce (page 350).

2 medium cucumbers, peeled, seeded, and sliced	2 tablespoons extra-virgin olive oil
1½ cups halved and thinly sliced radishes	2 teaspoons red wine vinegar
¼ cup fresh mint leaves, thinly sliced (optional)	5 ounces reduced-fat feta cheese, crumbled (1 cup)
2 tablespoons minced red onion	Salt and freshly ground black pepper

Combine cucumber, radishes, mint (if using), onion, oil, and vinegar in a large mixing bowl. Gently toss in feta, season to taste with salt and pepper, and serve.

Makes 4 (1½-cup) servings

NUTRITION AT A GLANCE

Per serving: 140 calories, 11 g fat, 3.5 g saturated fat, 8 g protein, 5 g carbohydrate, 1 g dietary fiber, 480 mg sodium

Turkey Salad with Pistachios and Grapes

PREP TIME: 10 minutes

Celery and nuts add crunch to this delectable warm-weather salad, and grapes add a hint of sweetness. Eat it with your favorite greens or stuff it into a whole-grain pita pocket for a tasty sandwich.

1½ pounds roast turkey or chicken, cut into ½-inch cubes

4 celery stalks, chopped

¾ cup grapes, sliced in half

⅓ cup shelled salted pistachios, roughly chopped

⅓ cup mayonnaise

¼ teaspoon salt

¼ teaspoon freshly ground black pepper

Combine turkey, celery, grapes, pistachios, mayonnaise, salt, and pepper in a large mixing bowl. Stir well to coat and refrigerate until ready to serve.

Makes 6 (1-cup) servings

NUTRITION AT A GLANCE

Per serving: 290 calories, 16 g fat, 2.5 g saturated fat, 30 g protein, 6 g carbohydrate, 0 g dietary fiber, 250 mg sodium

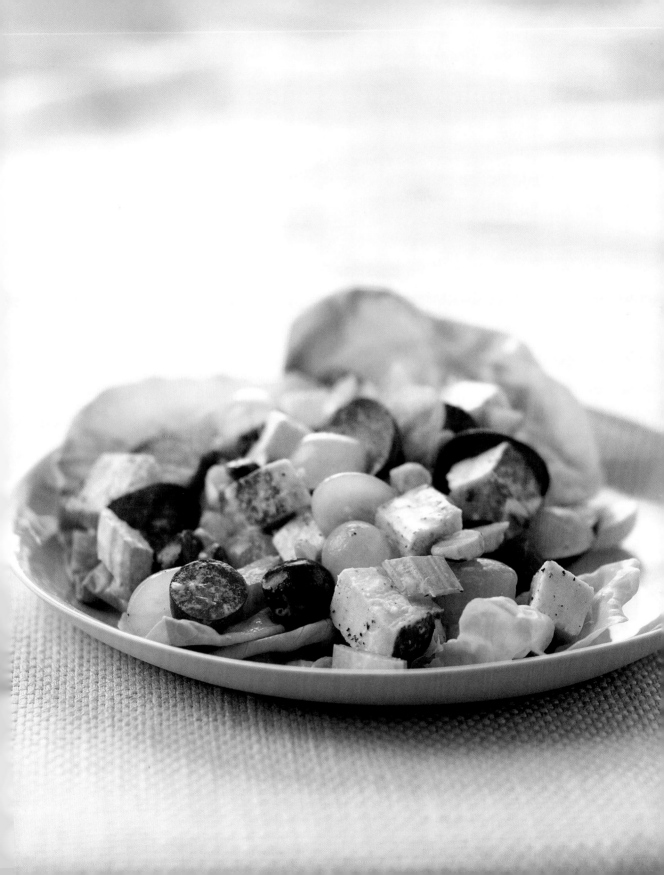

Simple Arugula Salad

PREP TIME: 5 minutes

This tasty, crisp salad pairs well with any dish.

> 1 (6-ounce) package arugula, torn into bite-size pieces (8 cups)
>
> 4 radishes, thinly sliced
>
> 2 tablespoons extra-virgin olive oil
>
> 1 tablespoon red wine vinegar
>
> Salt and freshly ground black pepper

Toss together arugula, radishes, oil, and vinegar in a large mixing bowl. Season with salt and pepper to taste and serve.

Makes 4 (2-cup) servings

NUTRITION AT A GLANCE

Per serving: 80 calories, 7 g fat, 1 g saturated fat, 1 g protein, 2 g carbohydrate, 0 g dietary fiber, 85 mg sodium

Moroccan Cabbage and Carrot Slaw

PREP TIME: 20 minutes

This tangy, spiced slaw makes a great salad or side for chicken, steak, or fish. Carrots are packed with fiber, iron, and the potent antioxidant beta-carotene. Use a food processor to shred veggies fast.

- ½ cup mayonnaise
- 2 tablespoons fresh lemon juice
- 2 scallions, thinly sliced
- 2 teaspoons granular sugar substitute
- 1 teaspoon ground cumin
- 1 (1- to 1½-pound) head green cabbage, shredded (4 to 5 cups)
- 3 medium carrots, shredded

  Salt and freshly ground black pepper

Whisk together mayonnaise, lemon juice, scallions, sugar substitute, and cumin in a large mixing bowl. Add cabbage and carrots and toss to combine. Season to taste with salt and pepper and refrigerate until ready to serve.

Makes 8 (¾-cup) servings

NUTRITION AT A GLANCE

Per serving: 140 calories, 11 g fat, 1.5 g saturated fat, 1 g protein, 9 g carbohydrate, 3 g dietary fiber, 160 mg sodium

Tricolor Salad

PREP TIME: 10 minutes

Peppery arugula and crisp Belgian endive and radicchio form this colorful, tasty Italian salad that's almost too pretty to eat.

2 anchovy fillets (optional)

1 garlic clove, minced

1 tablespoon balsamic vinegar

¼ teaspoon salt

¼ teaspoon freshly ground black pepper

3 tablespoons extra-virgin olive oil

1 (5-ounce) bag arugula (4 cups)

1 small head radicchio, cored and cut into ½-inch slices (3 cups)

2 small heads Belgian endive, cut into ½-inch slices (3 cups)

1 ounce Parmesan cheese, shaved

Place anchovies in a large mixing bowl; using 2 forks, mash into a paste. Add garlic, vinegar, salt, and pepper; mix well. Slowly whisk in oil.

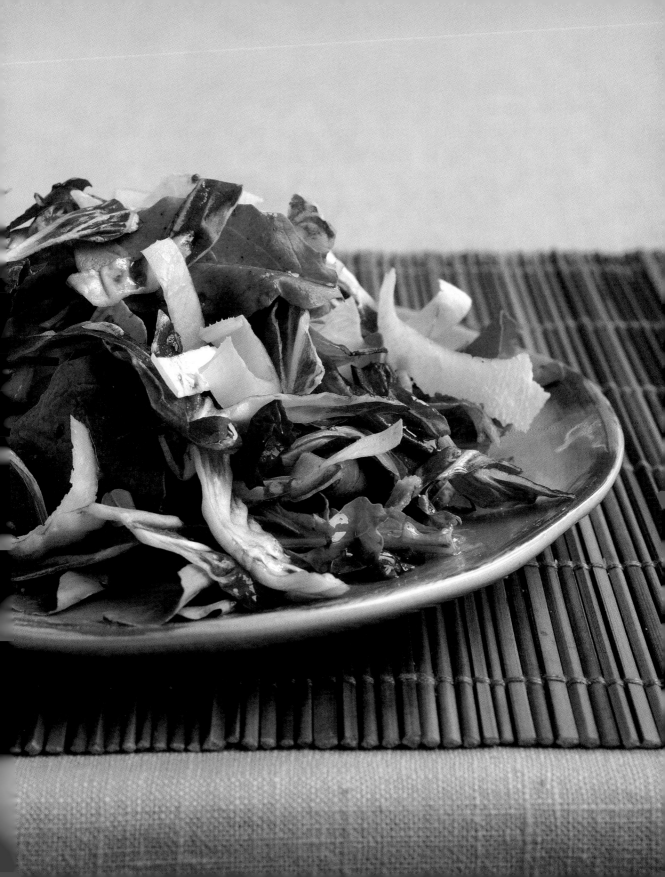

Add arugula, radicchio, and endive; toss to coat. Divide salad among 4 serving plates; sprinkle with cheese and serve.

Makes 4 (2-cup) servings

NUTRITION AT A GLANCE

Per serving: 150 calories, 13 g fat, 2.5 g saturated fat, 5 g protein, 6 g carbohydrate, 3 g dietary fiber, 280 mg sodium

Green Leaf, Pear, and Goat Cheese Salad

PREP TIME: 20 minutes

Ever since goat cheese became a common cooking ingredient, it seems to show up everywhere. Here, we mix it with freshly toasted walnuts, crisp fruity pear, and fresh leafy greens; the slightly smoky taste of the walnuts in this simple salad is a nice contrast to the creamy and delicious goat cheese.

⅓ cup walnuts

3 tablespoons extra-virgin olive oil

1 tablespoon fresh lemon juice

1 (¾-pound) head green leaf lettuce, torn into bite-size pieces (6 cups loosely packed)

½ Bosc pear, cored and thinly sliced

3 ounces plain reduced-fat soft goat cheese

Salt and freshly ground black pepper

Heat oven or toaster oven to 275°F. Spread walnuts on a baking tray and bake until fragrant and lightly browned, about 10 minutes. Roughly chop nuts.

Place oil, lemon juice, and a pinch of salt and pepper in a jar with a lid. Close tightly and shake vigorously to combine.

Place lettuce and pear slices in a mixing bowl. Season

with salt and pepper, add dressing, and toss. Divide among plates, sprinkle cheese and nuts on top, and serve.

Makes 4 (3-cup) servings

NUTRITION AT A GLANCE

Per serving: 200 calories, 18 g fat, 3.5 g saturated fat, 4 g protein, 7 g carbohydrate, 2 g dietary fiber, 190 mg sodium

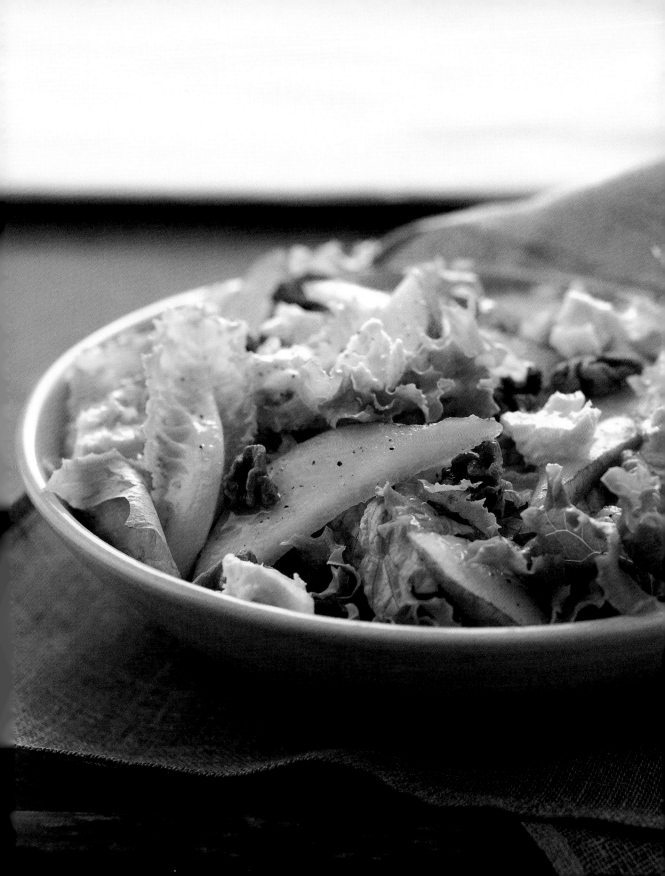

Turkey Antipasto Salad

PREP TIME: 10 minutes

We've turned a beloved Italian appetizer into a colorful and delicious salad that makes a satisfying meal for lunch or a light dinner. You can add other favorites, like a few olives or a tablespoon or two of canned beans per serving, as you like.

¼ cup extra-virgin olive oil

2 tablespoons red wine vinegar

1 tablespoon minced red onion

¼ teaspoon salt

⅛ teaspoon freshly ground black pepper

1 (1-pound) head romaine lettuce, chopped (8 cups)

¾ pound roasted turkey breast, sliced

2 large roasted red bell peppers, cut into thin strips

6 ounces marinated artichoke hearts (about 8 pieces)

4 ounces reduced-fat provolone, mozzarella, or muenster cheese, sliced or cubed

Place oil, vinegar, onion, salt, and pepper in a small glass jar. Close tightly and shake vigorously.

Arrange lettuce, turkey, bell peppers, artichokes, and cheese on 4 plates, antipasto style (separated into piles). Spoon dressing over the top and serve.

Makes 4 (2½-cup) servings

NUTRITION AT A GLANCE

Per serving: 360 calories, 22 g fat, 6 g saturated fat, 37 g protein, 10 g carbohydrate, 3 g dietary fiber, 480 mg sodium

Chicken Tahini Salad

PREP TIME: 20 minutes   **COOK TIME:** 5 minutes

A rich and tasty Middle Eastern staple, tahini is a thick, nutty paste made from ground sesame seeds. You'll find it in large supermarkets as well as health food and specialty stores.

Dressing:

> 6 ounces plain low-fat or fat-free yogurt
>
> ¼ cup well-stirred tahini
>
> 3 tablespoons fresh lemon juice
>
> Salt and freshly ground black pepper

Salad:

> 4 ounces snow peas, cut into thirds
>
> 1 (¾-pound) head napa cabbage, shredded (4 cups)
>
> 1½ pounds cooked chicken breast, cut into ½-inch cubes
>
> 2 scallions, thinly sliced
>
> ⅔ cup dry-roasted, unsalted cashews, roughly chopped

For the dressing: Whisk together yogurt, tahini, and lemon juice in a large mixing bowl; season to taste with salt and pepper.

For the salad: Bring a medium saucepan of salted water to a boil. Add snow peas and cook until crisp-tender, about 1 minute. Drain and run under cold water; pat dry.

Add snow peas, cabbage, chicken, scallions, and cashews to dressing; toss to combine and serve.

Makes 4 (2-cup) servings

NUTRITION AT A GLANCE

Per serving: 470 calories, 21 g fat, 4 g saturated fat, 50 g protein, 20 g carbohydrate, 3 g dietary fiber, 160 mg sodium

Shrimp and Celery Salad

PREP TIME: 15 minutes

Fresh lime, curry powder, and creamy sour cream make a zesty dressing for this refreshing summer salad. In later phases, spoon it onto toasted whole-grain bread for a heavenly open-faced sandwich.

- ½ cup reduced-fat sour cream
- ¼ cup mayonnaise
- 2 tablespoons fresh lime juice
- 1 tablespoon grated lime zest
- 1½ teaspoons curry powder
- ¼ teaspoon salt
- 1½ pounds peeled, deveined, and cooked medium fresh or frozen shrimp (thaw if frozen)
- 4 large celery stalks, thinly sliced
- 1 large cucumber, peeled, seeded, and thinly sliced

Whisk together sour cream, mayonnaise, lime juice, lime zest, curry powder, and salt in a large bowl. Add shrimp, celery, and cucumber; toss gently to coat. Refrigerate until ready to serve.

Makes 4 (1½-cup) servings

NUTRITION AT A GLANCE

Per serving: 330 calories, 17 g fat, 4.5 g saturated fat, 37 g protein, 6 g carbohydrate, 2 g dietary fiber, 670 mg sodium

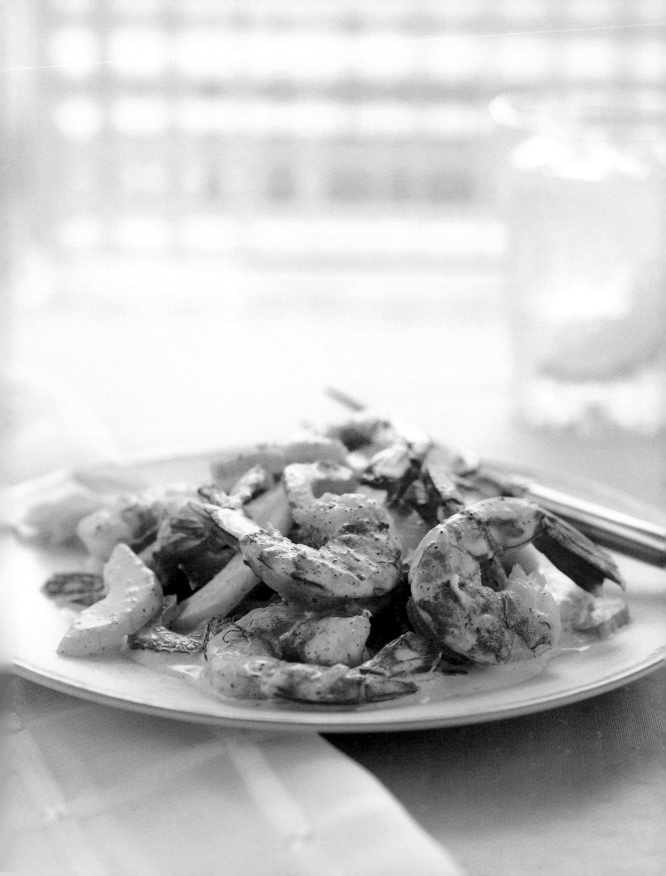

Brown Rice, Tomato, and Cucumber Salad

PREP TIME: 15 minutes   **COOK TIME: 25 minutes**

This refreshing salad offers a great way to use up leftover rice, but since the rice cooks up so quickly anyway, it's well worth preparing just for this recipe. Serve it as a main course, as a salad or, in smaller portions, as a side for steak, chicken, or fish.

½ cup whole-grain, quick-cooking brown rice (see page 14)

1 (¾-pound) head romaine or arugula, torn into bite-size pieces (6 cups)

1 medium cucumber, peeled, seeded, and sliced

1 plum tomato, diced

2 scallions, thinly sliced

3 tablespoons extra-virgin olive oil

1 tablespoon red wine vinegar

Salt and freshly ground black pepper

Cook rice according to package directions. Remove from heat, spread on a plate, and refrigerate for 10 minutes to cool.

Mix rice with romaine, cucumber, tomato, scallions, oil, and vinegar. Season with salt and pepper to taste and serve.

Makes 4 (2-cup) servings

NUTRITION AT A GLANCE

Per serving: 210 calories, 12 g fat, 1.5 g saturated fat, 3 g protein, 24 g carbohydrate, 3 g dietary fiber, 85 mg sodium

Red Leaf, Avocado, and Apple Salad

PREP TIME: 15 minutes

A grainy-mustard dressing makes an unlikely yet perfect marriage with the sweet and creamy flavors of the apple and the avocado.

2 tablespoons extra-virgin olive oil

2 teaspoons fresh lemon juice

½ teaspoon coarse-grain Dijon mustard

1 (1-pound) head red leaf lettuce, torn into bite-size pieces (8 cups)

1 avocado, pitted, peeled, and thinly sliced

½ Granny Smith apple, thinly sliced

Salt and freshly ground black pepper

Combine oil, lemon juice, and mustard in a jar. Add a pinch of salt and pepper, close tightly, and shake vigorously to combine.

Toss dressing with lettuce; add salt and pepper to taste. Distribute salad among plates, top with avocado and apple slices, and serve.

Makes 4 (2-cup) servings

NUTRITION AT A GLANCE

Per serving: 180 calories, 15 g fat, 2.5 g saturated fat, 3 g protein, 12 g carbohydrate, 5 g dietary fiber, 95 mg sodium

Cannellini Bean Salad

PREP TIME: 10 minutes

This quick, easy bean salad is great cold or at room temperature, making it a good take-along dish for work, the beach, or a potluck. Serve it as a side with grilled chicken or fish. You can substitute 2 or 3 tablespoons chopped fresh herbs for dried and try basil in place of oregano, if you wish.

- 2 tablespoons extra-virgin olive oil
- 1 tablespoon red wine vinegar
- 1 tablespoon minced red onion
- ¾ teaspoon dried oregano
- 2 medium cucumbers, peeled, seeded, and diced
- 1 (15-ounce) can cannellini beans, rinsed and drained
- 1 red bell pepper, finely diced

  Salt and freshly ground black pepper

Whisk together oil, vinegar, onion, and oregano in a large mixing bowl. Add cucumbers, beans, and bell pepper; toss to combine. Season with salt and pepper and serve.

Makes 4 (1-cup) servings

NUTRITION AT A GLANCE

Per serving: 180 calories, 8 g fat, 1 g saturated fat, 7 g protein, 22 g carbohydrate, 5 g dietary fiber, 80 mg sodium

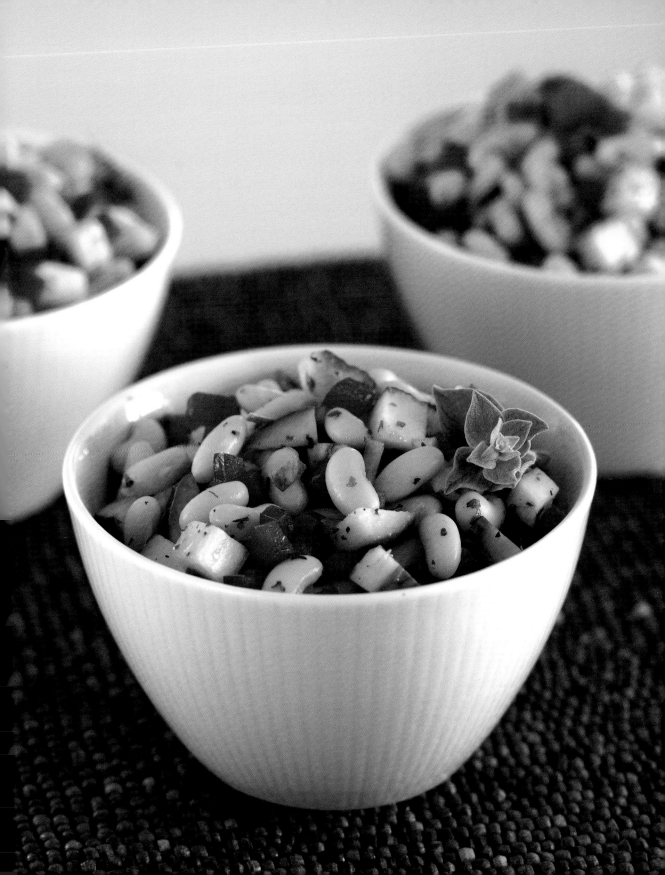

Cajun Chicken Salad

PREP TIME: 10 minutes

Our tangy yogurt dressing, combined with crisp lettuce, cools off this peppery flavor-packed salad. The dressing can do double duty as a fresh veggies dip, and you can use the salad as a sandwich filling in later phases. If you don't have Cajun seasoning, use a mix of any of the following: garlic powder, onion powder, cayenne pepper, mustard powder, black pepper, and celery salt.

- 1 small red onion
- ½ cup plain fat-free yogurt
- ½ teaspoon sugar-free Cajun seasoning
- 1 (1-pound) head romaine lettuce, cut into 1-inch slices (8 cups)
- 1 medium cucumber, peeled, seeded, and thinly sliced
- 4 (6-ounce) boneless, skinless chicken breasts, cooked and thinly sliced

  Salt and freshly ground black pepper

Mince enough onion to equal 1 tablespoon and thinly slice the rest into rings. Whisk together yogurt, Cajun seasoning, and minced onion in a large mixing bowl.

Add lettuce, cucumber, and onion slices and toss to combine; season to taste with salt and pepper. Arrange salad on plates and top with sliced chicken.

Makes 4 (3-cup) servings

NUTRITION AT A GLANCE

Per serving: 240 calories, 2.5 g fat, .5 g saturated fat, 42 g protein, 9 g carbohydrate, 3 g dietary fiber, 280 mg sodium

Spinach Salad with Grilled Chicken and Pomegranate Seeds

PREP TIME: 10 minutes   **COOK TIME: 20 minutes**

Pomegranates offer powerful antioxidants, as well as vitamins B_6 and C and potassium; they are available September through January. Freeze the seeds in a well-sealed container for up to a year so you can enjoy this colorful and delicious salad anytime.

¼ cup walnut pieces

1½ pounds boneless, skinless chicken breasts

3 tablespoons, plus 1 teaspoon extra-virgin olive oil, divided

3 tablespoons balsamic vinegar

1 garlic clove, minced

10 ounces baby spinach (8 cups)

1 pomegranate, seeded

Salt and freshly ground black pepper

Heat oven or toaster oven to 275°F. Lay walnuts in a single layer on a baking sheet and cook until fragrant and toasted, 8 to 10 minutes. Set aside to cool.

Toss chicken with 1 teaspoon oil and season with salt and pepper. Heat grill to medium-high or a grill pan over medium-high heat. Grill the chicken until no longer pink inside, about 4 minutes per side. Transfer to cutting board, cool slightly, and slice crosswise into ½-inch pieces.

Whisk together vinegar, remaining oil, and garlic in a large bowl; add the spinach and walnuts. Toss to coat, divide among 4 plates, top with chicken slices, and sprinkle with pomegranate seeds.

Makes 4 (3-cup) servings

NUTRITION AT A GLANCE

Per serving: 410 calories, 19 g fat, 2.5 g saturated fat, 43 g protein, 17 g carbohydrate, 4 g dietary fiber, 300 mg sodium

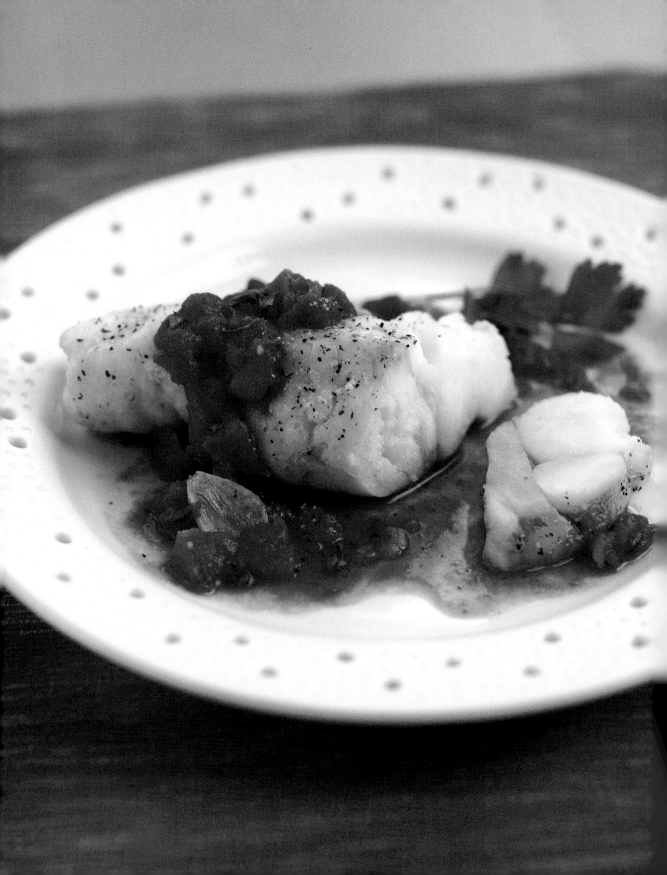

FISH AND SHELLFISH

Quick-cooking and highly nutritious, fish is a natural choice on the South Beach Diet. Salmon, mackerel, and sardines are particularly beneficial because they're high in omega-3 fatty acids; the former two also offer significant amounts of the antioxidant selenium and vitamins B_{12} and D. Most fish are excellent sources of lean protein, and all types offer heme iron, the form most readily absorbed by our bodies.

You can sauté, grill, roast, bake, broil, poach, or steam fish—each method requires little fat and is easy to master. If you enjoy bold flavors, try our Spanish Monkfish or the baked sea bass rubbed with chermoula. Milder options include delicious Seared Salmon with Zucchini. Fast favorites, like Shrimp Scampi served with a freshly tossed salad, make perfect weeknight meals.

◄ *Spanish Monkfish (page 200)*

Spanish Monkfish

PREP TIME: 5 minutes   **COOK TIME: 25 minutes**

Home cooks in Spain know that it's easy to put a quick and tasty meal on the table by using flavorful basics—garlic, tomatoes, parsley, and saffron—and simple technique. Following their philosophy and style, we created this delicious, no-fuss dish. Serve it with a salad or, in later phases, Nutty Brown Rice (page 421).

    1 tablespoon plus 2 teaspoons extra-virgin olive
      oil, divided

    2 garlic cloves, thinly sliced

    1 (14-ounce) can diced tomatoes

    ¼ teaspoon powdered saffron

  1½ pounds monkfish or halibut fillets

    2 tablespoons chopped fresh parsley

      Salt and freshly ground black pepper

Heat oven to 425°F.

Heat 2 teaspoons of the oil in a small saucepan over medium heat. Add garlic, reduce heat to medium-low, and cook 2 minutes. Add tomatoes with juice, saffron, and a pinch of salt and pepper. Simmer 20 minutes.

While sauce is cooking, brush fish with remaining oil and season well with salt and pepper. Bake until just opaque in the center, 12 to 15 minutes.

Add parsley to sauce, season to taste with salt and pepper, and remove from heat. Spoon over fish and serve.

Makes 4 servings

NUTRITION AT A GLANCE

Per serving: 200 calories, 8 g fat, 1.5 g saturated fat, 26 g protein, 5 g carbohydrate, 2 g dietary fiber, 230 mg sodium

Balsamic Glazed Salmon

PREP TIME: 5 minutes   **COOK TIME:** 12 minutes

Reducing balsamic vinegar (simmering it until it decreases in volume) turns it into a thick and flavorful glaze that, because of its sweet taste, pairs perfectly with rich salmon. Once you have this easy sauce mastered, you can try it on grilled steaks, chicken, or pork.

4 (6-ounce) salmon fillets

1 cup balsamic vinegar

2 teaspoons extra-virgin olive oil

1 teaspoon fresh lemon juice

Salt and freshly ground black pepper

Heat oven to 450°F.

Season salmon with salt and pepper; place in an ovenproof baking dish and bake until opaque throughout, 10 to 12 minutes.

While fish is cooking, place vinegar in a small saucepan. Cook over medium-high heat, stirring frequently, until reduced to $\frac{1}{3}$ cup, 8 to 10 minutes. Remove from heat, whisk in oil and lemon juice, and season with salt and pepper. Place salmon on serving plates and drizzle with glaze.

Makes 4 servings

NUTRITION AT A GLANCE

Per serving: 380 calories, 21 g fat, 4.5 g saturated fat, 34 g protein, 9 g carbohydrate, 0 g dietary fiber, 100 mg cholesterol, 190 mg sodium

Spiced Grouper with Mild Chile Purée

PREP TIME: 10 minutes   **COOK TIME: 15 minutes**

Mild chiles blend perfectly with warm cumin and zesty lime in a sauce that whips up in just minutes. Cod, snapper, and halibut also work well in this recipe.

Sauce:

> 1 (4-ounce) can whole green chiles, drained
>
> 2 tablespoons reduced-fat sour cream
>
> ¼ teaspoon salt

Fish:

> 1 tablespoon ground cumin
>
> ⅛ teaspoon cayenne pepper
>
> 4 (6-ounce) grouper fillets, about ½ inch thick
>
> 2 teaspoons extra-virgin olive oil
>
> 1 lime, cut into wedges
>
> Salt and freshly ground black pepper

For the sauce: Chop chiles, sour cream, and salt in a food processor until well blended.

For the fish: Mix cumin and cayenne together and rub into both sides of fish. Season fish well with salt and pepper.

Heat 1 teaspoon of the oil in a large nonstick skillet over medium-high heat, add 2 grouper fillets and cook until opaque and tender, about 3 minutes per side. Repeat with remaining oil and fish. Squeeze lime over fish and serve hot with sauce.

Makes 4 servings

NUTRITION AT A GLANCE

Per serving: 200 calories, 5 g fat, 1.5 g saturated fat, 34 g protein, 3 g carbohydrate, 0 g dietary fiber, 400 mg sodium

Ginger Steamed Red Snapper

PREP TIME: 5 minutes   **COOK TIME:** 25 minutes

Steaming is a great no-fat way to prepare a delicate fish like red snapper—but you don't have to give up on flavor. Adding chunks of fresh ginger and a touch of mirin or rice wine (page 38) to the steaming liquid gives this dish a delicious Asian flair. Serve it with Chinese-Style Broccoli (page 420). If you don't have mirin on hand, use our substitution below.

- 1 tablespoon sesame seeds
- 1 (5-inch) piece fresh ginger
- ¼ cup mirin or rice wine (or ¼ cup white wine plus 1 tablespoon granular sugar substitute)
- 4 (6-ounce) red snapper fillets
- 8 scallions, cut in half crosswise and thinly sliced lengthwise
- 2 teaspoons dark sesame oil

  Salt and freshly ground black pepper

Toast sesame seeds in a small skillet over low heat, stirring frequently, until fragrant and golden, about 3 minutes.

Finely grate 1 tablespoon ginger and roughly chop the rest to fill about a ¼ cup measure. Place chopped ginger in a large saucepan and cover with water to reach 2 inches. Add vinegar and bring to a simmer.

Season snapper with grated ginger, salt, and pepper. Place in steamer insert, add scallions, cover, and steam until flesh flakes easily, about 10 minutes.

Serve hot, drizzled with oil and topped with sesame seeds.

Makes 4 servings

NUTRITION AT A GLANCE

Per serving: 240 calories, 5 g fat, 1.5 g saturated fat, 35 g protein, 4 g carbohydrate, 1 g dietary fiber, 160 mg sodium

Fresh Tuna Salad with Simple Lemon Dijon

PREP TIME: 10 minutes   **COOK TIME: 5 minutes**

Crisp Bibb lettuce, tangy lemon, and sweet peas give this tasty fresh tuna salad a spring-like flavor. It seems fancy, yet takes just minutes to prepare!

- 2 tablespoons fresh lemon juice
- 1 tablespoon minced red onion
- 1 teaspoon Dijon mustard
- ¼ cup plus 2 teaspoons canola oil, divided
- 1 pound fresh tuna, about 1 inch thick
- 1 (8-ounce) head Bibb or Boston lettuce, torn into bite-size pieces (4 to 5 cups)
- ½ cup frozen peas, thawed
- Salt and freshly ground black pepper

Whisk together lemon juice, onion, and mustard in a mixing bowl. Slowly whisk in ¼ cup of the oil. Season to taste with salt and pepper.

Season tuna with salt and pepper. Heat remaining oil in a large skillet over medium-high heat. Cook tuna 1½ minutes per side for medium-rare or to desired doneness. Transfer to a cutting board.

Divide lettuce among serving plates and sprinkle with peas. Slice tuna and divide among salads; drizzle with dressing and serve.

Makes 4 servings

NUTRITION AT A GLANCE

Per serving: 290 calories, 18 g fat, 1.5 g saturated fat, 28 g protein, 5 g carbohydrate, 1 g dietary fiber, 150 mg sodium

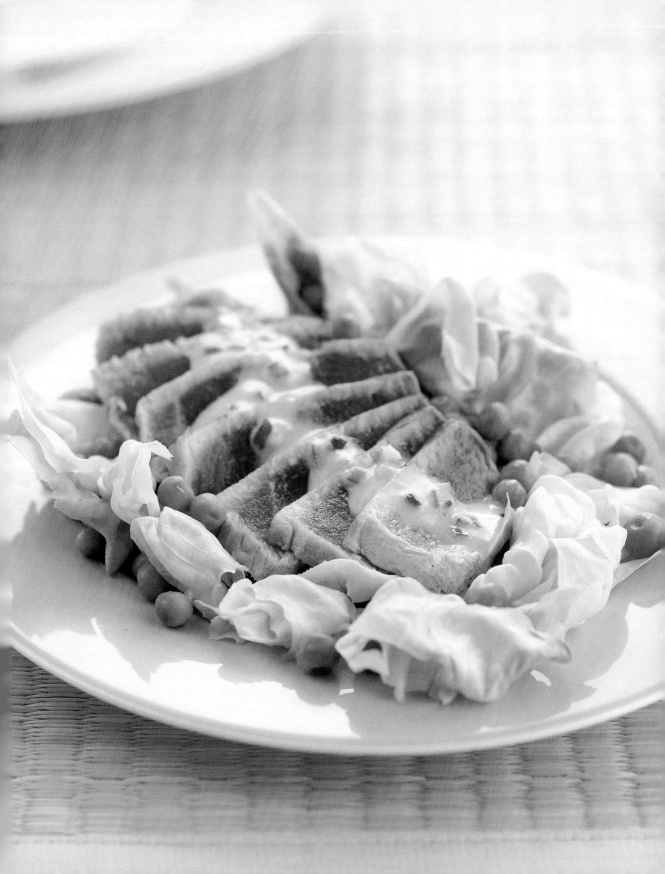

Baked Sea Bass with Chermoula

PREP TIME: 5 minutes   **COOK TIME:** 15 minutes

Chermoula is a flavorful Moroccan condiment, most often used in fish dishes although it's also fantastic on chicken, beef, and lamb. If sea bass is unavailable, try salmon, monkfish, or cod. You can use parsley in place of cilantro— or a mix of both.

1 bunch cilantro, leaves and stems intact

4 garlic cloves, peeled

2 teaspoons ground cumin

¼ teaspoon red pepper flakes

¼ cup extra-virgin olive oil

¼ cup fresh lemon juice

4 (6-ounce) sea bass fillets

Salt and freshly ground black pepper

Heat oven to 450°F.

Chop cilantro, garlic, cumin, red pepper flakes, and a large pinch of salt in a food processor; with the machine running, drizzle in oil and lemon juice.

Season both sides of fish with salt and pepper. Spread one-quarter of the chermoula in an ovenproof baking dish, lay fish on top, and cover evenly with remaining chermoula. Bake until fish is opaque and tender, 12 to 15 minutes. Serve hot.

Makes 4 servings

NUTRITION AT A GLANCE

Per serving: 310 calories, 18 g fat, 3 g saturated fat, 32 g protein, 3 g carbohydrate, 0 g dietary fiber, 190 mg sodium

Mahi Mahi with Citrus

PREP TIME: 5 minutes
COOK TIME: 20 minutes (includes marinating)

Mahi mahi is a sturdy fish that stands up well to pan or grill cooking. Whatever way you choose to cook it, the tangy citrus and toasty garlic flavors will come through beautifully. Turn leftovers into Mahi Mahi Salad by adding chopped cucumber and scallion and a drop or two of mayo; in later phases, you can serve it on a crisp slice of whole-grain toast.

2 tablespoons extra-virgin olive oil

1 tablespoon fresh lemon juice

1 tablespoon fresh lime juice

1 garlic clove, minced

½ teaspoon dried thyme

4 (6-ounce) skinless mahi mahi fillets, about ¾ inch thick

Salt and freshly ground black pepper

Whisk together oil, lemon juice, lime juice, garlic, thyme, and salt and pepper to taste. Place fish in a shallow dish, drizzle with citrus mixture, turn to coat, and marinate at room temperature for 10 minutes.

Heat grill pan or nonstick skillet over medium-high heat. Add fish and cook 3 to 4 minutes per side. Serve hot.

Makes 4 servings

NUTRITION AT A GLANCE

Per serving: 210 calories, 8 g fat, 1.5 g saturated fat, 32 g protein, 1 g carbohydrate, 0 g dietary fiber, 220 mg sodium

Halibut with Tapenade in Parchment

PREP TIME: 5 minutes

COOK TIME: 25 minutes (includes preparing packets)

These packets are opened at the table, where hot steam rises to reveal the tender, olive-cloaked fish. This dish seems fancy but is surprisingly easy to prepare. If halibut is unavailable, try salmon, flounder, or orange roughy. You can also try different vegetables, like roasted red pepper, zucchini, or even shaved fennel. The added bonus: Cleanup is a breeze.

2 tablespoons extra-virgin olive oil

2 tablespoons fresh lemon juice

2 medium tomatoes, diced

4 (6-ounce) halibut fillets, about 1 inch thick

4 teaspoons olive tapenade (from a jar)

Salt and freshly ground black pepper

Special equipment:

4 (15-inch-square) pieces parchment paper

4 (8-inch) pieces kitchen string

Arrange rack in lower third of oven and heat to 425°F.
Place oil, lemon juice, ½ teaspoon salt, and
¼ teaspoon pepper in a jar with a lid. Close tightly and shake vigorously to combine. Divide tomato equally onto the center of each piece of parchment paper; season with salt and pepper. Season halibut lightly on

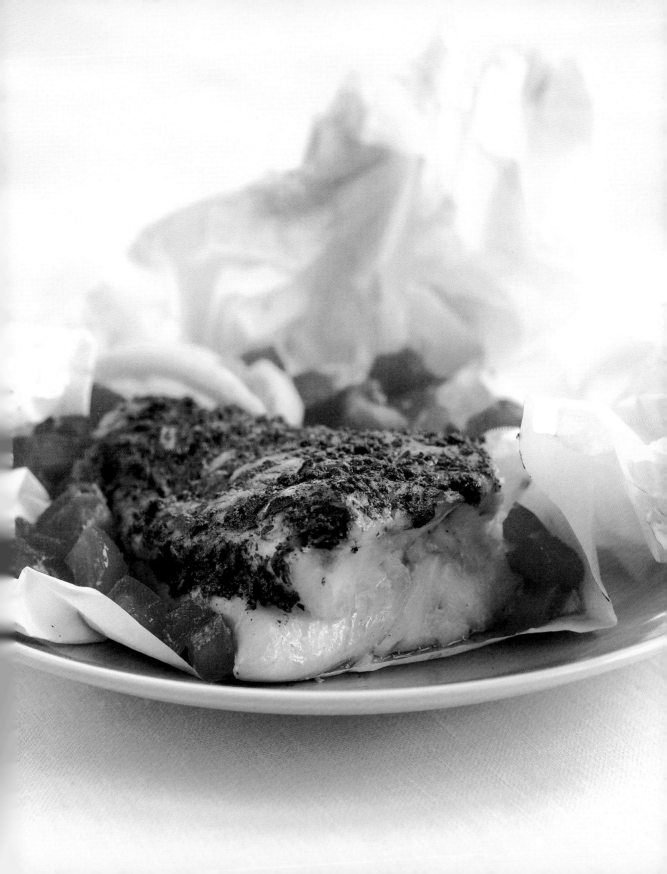

both sides with salt and pepper; place 1 piece on top of each mound of tomatoes. Spread 1 teaspoon of tapenade on top of each piece of fish, then drizzle each with 1 tablespoon of the lemon juice mixture. Gather up sides of parchment over fish (one at a time) and tie each piece closed with kitchen string, leaving as much air inside the packets and around the fish as possible.

Place packets on a baking sheet and bake until fish is cooked through, 13 to 15 minutes (you can open one of the packets to check for doneness). Transfer packets to plates and serve, snipping string and opening at the table.

Makes 4 servings

NUTRITION AT A GLANCE

Per serving: 270 calories, 11 g fat, 1.5 g saturated fat, 36 g protein, 4 g carbohydrate, 1 g dietary fiber, 230 mg sodium

Seared Salmon with Zucchini

PREP TIME: 5 minutes   **COOK TIME: 20 minutes**

Filled with protein and rich in A and B vitamins and omega-3s, salmon is one of the healthiest fish you can eat. This dish illustrates its ability to deliver big flavor—even with a very simple recipe.

- 2 tablespoons extra-virgin olive oil, divided
- ½ small red onion, minced
- 2 large zucchini, thinly sliced into rounds
- 4 (6-ounce) salmon fillets
- Salt and freshly ground black pepper

Heat 1 tablespoon of the oil in a large skillet over medium-high heat. Add onion and cook until softened, about 3 minutes. Add zucchini and cook until softened and lightly browned, 2 to 3 minutes. Cover and cook 2 minutes more. Season vegetables well with salt and pepper; transfer to a plate and cover loosely with foil to keep warm.

Season salmon with salt and pepper. Heat remaining oil in the same skillet over medium-high heat. Add salmon, skin side down, and cook until lightly browned, 3 minutes per side. Serve with vegetables.

Makes 4 servings

NUTRITION AT A GLANCE

Per serving: 400 calories, 26 g fat, 5 g saturated fat, 36 g protein, 6 g carbohydrate, 2 g dietary fiber, 190 mg sodium

Sardines with Lemon and Hot Sauce

PREP TIME: 5 minutes

Get a burst of omega-3s with this zesty sardine dish. If fresh sardines are available at your local fish market, try them in place of canned; just season them with salt and pepper, grill 2 minutes per side, and serve with hot sauce and lots of lemon wedges for squeezing. Serve two fresh sardines per person.

- 3 tablespoons extra-virgin olive oil
- 2 tablespoons fresh lemon juice
- ½ teaspoon Dijon mustard
- 3 (3.75-ounce) cans sardines packed in water, drained
- Hot pepper sauce
- 10 ounces spring mix or mesclun greens (8 to 10 cups)
- Salt and freshly ground black pepper

Whisk together oil, lemon juice, mustard, and a pinch of salt and pepper in a large mixing bowl. Lay sardines on a plate and drizzle with 1 tablespoon of the dressing; sprinkle with pepper and a dash or two of hot pepper sauce.

Add greens to the bowl; toss to combine. Divide salad among plates, top with sardines, and serve with extra hot sauce.

Makes 4 servings

NUTRITION AT A GLANCE

Per serving: 310 calories, 23 g fat, 5 g saturated fat, 22 g protein, 3 g carbohydrate, 1 g dietary fiber, 860 mg sodium

Grilled Pepper Tuna

PREP TIME: 3 minutes   **COOK TIME: 10 minutes**

Just about as simple as it gets but a tried-and-true favorite, this delectable tuna melts in your mouth. Serve it with Tricolor Salad (page 178).

   1 teaspoon black peppercorns

   1 tablespoon extra-virgin olive oil

   4 (6-ounce) tuna steaks, about 1 inch thick

   1 teaspoon grated lemon zest (optional)

    Salt

Heat grill or grill pan to medium-high. Lay peppercorns flat on work surface and place a clean skillet on top. Press down to crush peppercorns a few at a time until all peppercorns are cracked. Rub oil over steaks and season with salt, cracked pepper, and lemon zest, if using.

    Grill tuna 2½ minutes per side for rare, 3 minutes per side for medium-rare, and 3½ minutes per side to be cooked through. Serve hot, sliced or whole.

Makes 4 servings

NUTRITION AT A GLANCE

Per serving: 220 calories, 5 g fat, 1 g saturated fat, 40 g protein, 0 g carbohydrate, 0 g dietary fiber, 135 mg sodium

Shrimp Scampi

PREP TIME: 10 minutes   **COOK TIME:** 8 minutes

This quick classic is a sure bet for garlic and butter lovers. Serve it alongside Eggless Caesar Salad (page 161) or over whole-wheat pasta or brown rice in later phases.

- 1½ pounds fresh or thawed frozen shrimp, peeled and deveined
- 3 tablespoons trans-fat-free margarine
- 4 garlic cloves, minced
- ¼ cup fresh lemon juice
- 3 tablespoons chopped fresh parsley
- ⅛ teaspoon red pepper flakes
- Salt and freshly ground black pepper

Rinse shrimp under cold water and pat dry well with a paper towel. Season with salt and pepper.

Heat margarine and garlic in a large skillet over medium heat until melted and bubbling, 1 to 2 minutes. Add shrimp and stir to coat with margarine.

Add lemon juice, parsley, and red pepper flakes; cook, stirring occasionally, until shrimp are pink, about 2 minutes; do not overcook or the shrimp will be tough. Remove from heat, season with salt and pepper, and serve hot.

Makes 4 servings

NUTRITION AT A GLANCE

Per serving: 230 calories, 10 g fat, 2.5 g saturated fat, 31 g protein, 4 g carbohydrate, 0 g dietary fiber, 360 mg sodium

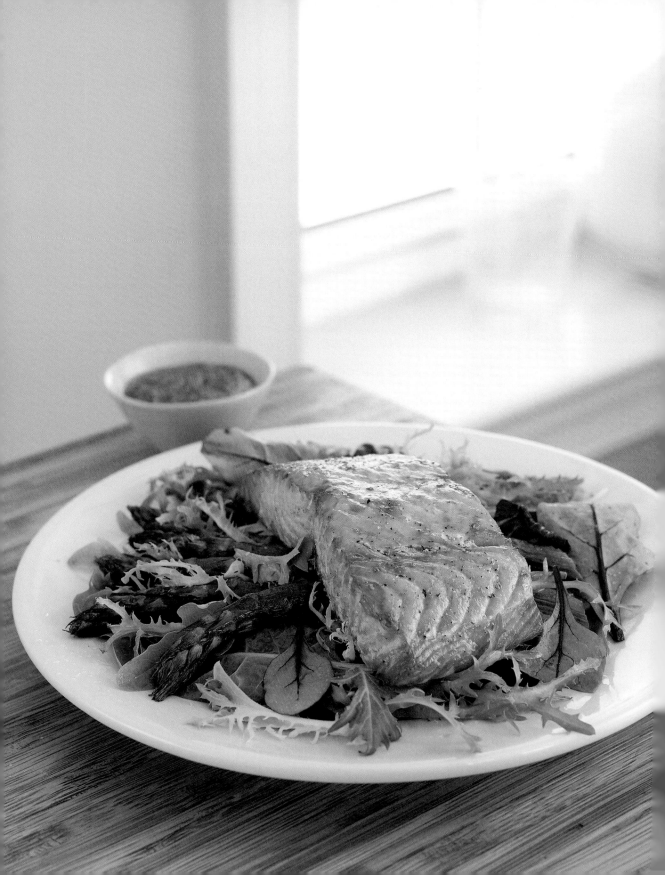

Warm Salmon and Asparagus Salad

PREP TIME: 10 minutes   **COOK TIME:** 20 minutes

Roasting asparagus imparts a deep, complex flavor that gives the ordinary steamed version a run for its money. This elegant dish is great for guests, but it's also quick enough for a simple weeknight meal.

- 2 pounds asparagus, ends trimmed
- 2 tablespoons plus 2 teaspoons extra-virgin olive oil, divided, plus extra for baking dish
- 4 (6-ounce) salmon fillets
- 2 tablespoons coarse-grain Dijon mustard
- 1 tablespoon white wine vinegar
- 5 ounces mesclun greens (6 cups)
    Salt and freshly ground black pepper

Heat oven to 450°F.

Place asparagus in a single layer in a baking pan; drizzle with 2 teaspoons of the oil, season with salt and pepper, and turn to coat. Bake until lightly browned, about 20 minutes.

While asparagus is roasting, season salmon with salt and pepper. Lightly brush a baking dish with oil, add salmon, and bake until fish flakes easily with a fork, 10 to 12 minutes.

Place mustard, vinegar, remaining oil, ¼ teaspoon salt, and ⅛ teaspoon pepper in a glass jar with a lid.

Close tightly and shake vigorously to combine; adjust seasoning if necessary.

Combine greens and 2 tablespoons of the dressing in a mixing bowl; toss to coat. Drizzle remaining dressing over the fish and serve with asparagus and greens.

Makes 4 servings

NUTRITION AT A GLANCE

Per serving: 500 calories, 33 g fat, 6 g saturated fat, 40 g protein, 11 g carbohydrate, 5 g dietary fiber, 360 mg sodium

Cod with Artichokes and Basil

PREP TIME: 5 minutes   **COOK TIME:** 15 minutes

Marinated artichokes are a great convenience product because they provide concentrated flavor and a delicious liquid, which can also be used to flavor a dish. Together with aromatic basil, they are the perfect foil for flaky, light cod. You can also try pollock, haddock, snapper, or turbot for this recipe.

1½ pounds cod fillet

1 tablespoon plus 1½ teaspoons extra-virgin olive oil

1 tablespoon dried basil

10 ounces marinated artichoke hearts (about 12 pieces), plus 1 tablespoon liquid from jar

Salt and freshly ground black pepper

Heat oven to 450°F.

Place cod in an ovenproof baking dish, brush with oil, sprinkle with basil, and season with salt and pepper. Arrange artichoke hearts around fish and drizzle with artichoke liquid.

Bake until fish is opaque and just flakes with a fork, 12 to 14 minutes. Remove from oven and serve hot.

Makes 4 servings

NUTRITION AT A GLANCE

Per serving: 250 calories, 10 g fat, 1 g saturated fat, 33 g protein, 8 g carbohydrate, 3 g dietary fiber, 430 mg sodium

Baked Mackerel Fillets

PREP TIME: 5 minutes   COOK TIME: 20 minutes

A cousin of tuna, mackerel is a delicious oily fish that provides substantial benefits, including impressive amounts of omega-3s, vitamin B_{12}, and the antioxidant selenium. Tomatoes and olives add great flavor and balance the fish's rich taste.

- 4 (6-ounce) mackerel fillets
- 1 tablespoon extra-virgin olive oil
- ½ teaspoon dried oregano
- Pinch red pepper flakes
- ⅓ cup black olives, pitted and sliced
- 1 large garlic clove, thinly sliced
- 1 (14.5-ounce) can stewed tomatoes, drained and roughly chopped
- Salt and freshly ground black pepper

Heat oven to 375°F.

Rub mackerel with oil and season with salt and pepper. Place in an ovenproof baking dish and season with oregano and red pepper flakes. Top with olives and garlic, then cover with tomatoes. Sprinkle with salt and pepper and bake until fish flakes with a fork, about 20 minutes.

Makes 4 servings

NUTRITION AT A GLANCE

Per serving: 420 calories, 28 g fat, 6 g saturated fat, 33 g protein, 6 g carbohydrate, 2 g dietary fiber, 530 mg sodium

Crispy Trout with Lemon-Caper Sauce

PREP TIME: 15 minutes   **COOK TIME: 10 minutes**

The secret to a deliciously crispy trout is to rinse and then pat the fish dry completely before brushing it with oil and cooking it in a hot pan. Our sauce—made with tangy lemon juice, piquant capers, and trans-fat-free margarine—is the perfect foil for the tender, flaky fish.

- 4 tablespoons trans-fat-free margarine, melted
- 1 tablespoon fresh lemon juice
- 1 tablespoon capers, drained and rinsed
- 4 (5- to 6-ounce) trout fillets, skin on
- 1½ teaspoons canola oil, plus extra for brushing fish

  Salt and freshly ground black pepper

Whisk margarine, lemon juice, and capers together in a mixing bowl until smooth.

Rinse trout under cold water and pat dry well with paper towels. Brush with oil and season with salt and pepper.

Heat oil in a large nonstick skillet over medium-high heat until rippling but not smoking. Add trout, skin side down (in batches if necessary), and cook for 3 minutes; turn and cook 1 minute longer. Remove from pan, top with lemon sauce, and serve hot.

Makes 4 servings

NUTRITION AT A GLANCE

Per serving: 320 calories, 21 g fat, 4.5 g saturated fat, 30 g protein, 0 g carbohydrate, 0 g dietary fiber, 300 mg sodium

Steamed Halibut with Bell Pepper and Summer Squash

PREP TIME: 5 minutes   **COOK TIME: 10 minutes**

This easy meal cooks in just one pan, making for a no-fuss cleanup. Hake and cod are good substitutes for halibut, if you want a change of pace.

4	(6-ounce) halibut fillets, about ¾ inch thick at thickest part
1	orange bell pepper, cut into thin strips
1	medium yellow squash, cut into ⅛-inch, half-moon slices
2	tablespoons extra-virgin olive oil
2	tablespoons fresh lemon juice
1½	teaspoons Dijon mustard
	Salt and freshly ground black pepper

Fill bottom part of a steamer with 1 inch of water; bring to boil.

Season fish with salt and pepper and arrange in the steamer basket. Reduce to a rapid simmer, and cover with a lid. After fish has steamed for 3 minutes, arrange bell pepper and squash on top and around fish. Steam until fish is opaque and vegetables are tender, for a total of 6 to 8 minutes.

While fish and vegetables are cooking, whisk together oil, lemon juice, and mustard; add a pinch of salt and pepper.

Serve fish and vegetables hot, spooning sauce over the top.

Makes 4 servings

NUTRITION AT A GLANCE

Per serving: 270 calories, 11 g fat, 1.5 g saturated fat, 36 g protein, 4 g carbohydrate, 1 g dietary fiber, 190 mg sodium

Spicy Mussels with Tomato and Basil

PREP TIME: 5 minutes   **COOK TIME: 12 minutes**

Mussels—low in fat, high in protein, and rich in vitamin B$_{12}$ and omega-3 fatty acids—are the unsung heroes of quick (and cheap) eats in the seafood world. They pop open within minutes and pair well with all kinds of flavors. Serve them with a green salad and a big empty bowl for shells.

To clean mussels, simply run them under cold water, scrubbing gently with a vegetable brush. Discard any with broken shells and any with shells that remain open after being lightly tapped. As you go, pull off and discard the "beard" (the weedy piece that sometimes remains attached to the shell).

2 tablespoons extra-virgin olive oil

1 small onion, chopped

3 garlic cloves, minced

1 teaspoon dried basil

¼ teaspoon red pepper flakes

¾ cup white wine

¼ cup water

1 cup canned crushed tomatoes

4 pounds mussels, scrubbed and beards removed

Heat oil in a 6- to 8-quart heavy saucepan or Dutch oven over medium-high heat. Add onion, garlic, basil, and red pepper flakes. Cook, stirring occasionally, for 3 minutes, reducing heat if onions begin to brown.

Add wine and water, increase heat to high, bring to a boil, and cook 1 minute. Add tomatoes and mussels; cover and cook until mussels open, 6 to 8 minutes. Serve hot.

Makes 4 servings

NUTRITION AT A GLANCE

Per serving: 370 calories, 14 g fat, 2.5 g saturated fat, 37 g protein, 16 g carbohydrate, 0 g dietary fiber, 590 mg sodium

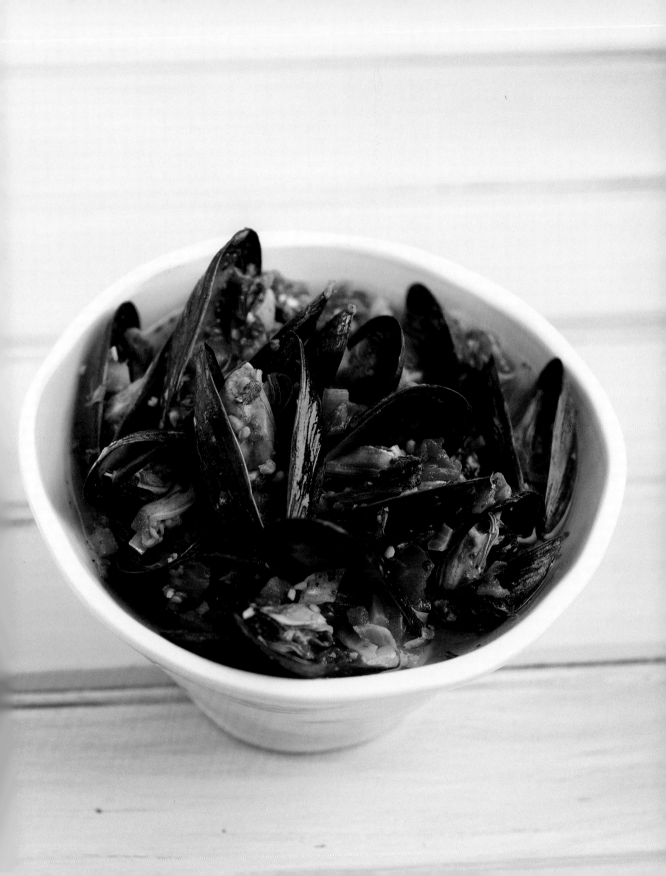

Shrimp Stir-Fry

PREP TIME: 15 minutes   **COOK TIME:** 10 minutes

Fresh ginger and garlic, plus a vibrant mixture of vegetables and tender shrimp, give this stir-fry big flavor and color. Make sure you have all the veggies prepared before you start to cook. Once you're ready, this dish cooks up in less than 10 minutes. If you can find cut packaged stir-fry vegetables at the supermarket, your prep time will be finished in a flash!

- 4 teaspoons canola oil, divided
- 2 tablespoons plus 1½ teaspoons low-sodium soy sauce, divided
- 3 garlic cloves, minced
- 1½ pounds medium peeled and deveined fresh or thawed frozen shrimp
- 2 tablespoons minced fresh ginger
- 8 ounces white mushrooms, quartered
- 4 scallions, cut into 1-inch pieces
- 1 large bell pepper, any color, cut into thin strips
- 8 ounces snow peas, strings removed
- ¼ teaspoon red pepper flakes

Whisk together 2 teaspoons of the oil, 1½ teaspoons of the soy sauce, and garlic in a large bowl; add shrimp and toss to coat.

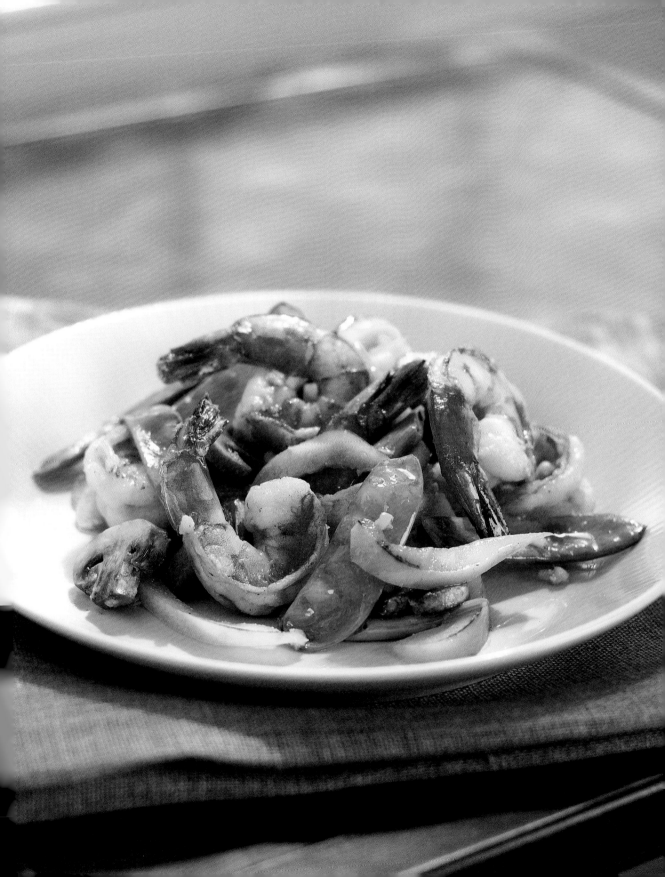

Lightly coat a large skillet or wok with cooking spray and heat over high heat. Add shrimp and cook until pink, 2 minutes. Transfer to a plate.

Heat remaining oil in the same skillet over high heat; add ginger and cook 30 seconds. Add mushrooms, scallions, bell pepper, snow peas, and red pepper flakes and cook until vegetables are crisp-tender, about 4 minutes. Stir in shrimp and remaining soy sauce and toss to combine. Serve hot.

Makes 4 (2-cup) servings

NUTRITION AT A GLANCE

Per serving: 280 calories, 8 g fat, 1 g saturated fat, 38 g protein, 13 g carbohydrate, 2 g dietary fiber, 600 mg sodium

Cod Chowder

PREP TIME: 5 minutes   **COOK TIME:** 35 minutes
(including standing time)

This buttery New England–style chowder does need to stand for a little bit before serving; we've speeded up prep time by cooking the fish in one piece.

  1 tablespoon trans-fat-free margarine

  3 slices turkey bacon, cut into ½-inch pieces

  1 large turnip, peeled and cut into ½-inch dice

  1 small onion, chopped

  3 celery stalks, chopped

  1 teaspoon dried thyme

16 ounces (2 cups) bottled clam juice, fish stock, or lower-sodium chicken broth

1¾ cups water

  1 cup fat-free half-and-half

1½ pounds skinless cod or haddock fillets, at least 1 inch thick, pinbones removed

   Salt and freshly ground black pepper

Heat margarine in a wide saucepan or Dutch oven over medium heat. Add turkey bacon and cook until browned, about 5 minutes. Remove with a slotted spoon and drain on paper towels.

   Add turnip, onion, celery, and thyme to the same pan. Cook over medium heat for 5 minutes. Add clam juice and water. Bring to a boil; reduce to a simmer, and cook for 5 minutes. Stir in half-and-half and reserved bacon.

Add fish, pushing vegetables to the side to allow fish to be mostly covered by liquid; bring back to a simmer and cook for 5 minutes. Cover, remove from heat, and allow chowder to stand for 10 minutes (fish will finish cooking during this time). Using a wooden spoon, gently break fish up into chunks. Season chowder with salt and pepper to taste and serve hot.

Makes 4 (2-cup) entrée servings or 8 (1-cup) appetizer servings

NUTRITION AT A GLANCE

Per entreé serving: 250 calories, 7 g fat, 2 g saturated fat, 35 g protein, 12 g carbohydrate, 2 g dietary fiber, 90 mg cholesterol, 700 mg sodium

MY SOUTH BEACH DIET

I believe the South Beach Diet saved my life.

We middle-aged, African-American women tend to put on the pounds and keep them on. We develop diabetes, heart disease, and high cholesterol—and I was in danger of all of these things, having gained 70 pounds since getting married 12 years ago. I'd tried everything: a 3-day cabbage soup diet, counting points, eating pre-packaged foods, calorie counting, fat counting, even eating nothing but a whole boiled chicken for a weekend. When my doctor suggested I lose weight and increase my exercise level, a friend of mine told me about the South Beach Diet. I did some research—and liked what I discovered.

The diet was surprisingly easy and consisted of all the foods I like. And, believe me, I like to eat! I started on South Beach just after New Year's, at 236 pounds. My biggest challenge was convincing my husband to join me. I knew from experience that success depended upon both of us being on the same diet, so I purchased The South Beach Diet book and started reading the menus and recipes to him. He decided that everything sounded good, and that the recipes didn't seem particularly "diet" to him. All of the recipes were easy to understand and prepare; the food was delicious and kept up our tradition of eating well-seasoned, flavorful dishes. I never had to make a separate "diet meal" for myself, and it was so simple to prepare the lunches and take them to work.

The first week's weight loss was phenomenal, and it convinced me that the South Beach Diet really works! Another encouraging factor was that changing my diet seems to have greatly reduced my persistent sinus problems and allergies. Plus, my husband and two teenage children love that I lost weight—and my husband has lost 38 pounds along with me.

I reached 178 pounds just 5 months after I started and have the pictures to prove it! Now, I am using the skills that I learned to maintain that weight, and I plan to go for the final 40 pounds very soon. And I'm having so much fun! I had stopped going out socially when I was bigger, but recently I went to a party where a friend who had not seen me for a while gushed that I looked "stunning."

I love the South Beach Diet, and I believe it saved my life. All I can say is: Thank you, thank you, thank you!!!

—KAREN W., ATLANTA, GEORGIA

Barbecued Salmon

PREP TIME: 5 minutes   **COOK TIME:** 10 minutes

The South Beach Barbecue Sauce is one of our favorite condiments. It's high in flavor and low in sugar—a hard-to-find combination in most store-bought brands. The rich texture of salmon is a perfect match.

> 4 (6-ounce) salmon fillets
>
> ½ cup South Beach Barbecue Sauce, divided (page 309)
>
> Vegetable oil, for grill
>
> Salt and freshly ground black pepper

Heat grill or grill pan to medium-high. Season fish with salt and pepper and generously brush top with ¼ cup of the barbecue sauce.

Brush grill with oil. Place fish, sauce side down, on grill; cook for 3 minutes. Brush top with the remaining sauce, flip, and cook an additional 3 to 4 minutes. Remove from grill. Serve warm.

Makes 4 servings

NUTRITION AT A GLANCE

Per serving: 330 calories, 20 g fat, 4 g saturated fat, 34 g protein, 2 g carbohydrate, 1 g dietary fiber, 330 mg sodium

Spaghetti with White Clam Sauce

PREP TIME: 10 minutes   **COOK TIME:** 15 minutes

A few ordinary pantry staples and presto! A tasty, steaming pasta—tossed with a creamy, garlicky clam sauce and fresh Parmesan—is on the table in no time. Reserved juices from canned clams give the sauce a deep, rich flavor.

    8 ounces whole-wheat spaghetti

    1 tablespoon extra-virgin olive oil

    6 garlic cloves, minced

    3 (6½-ounce) cans chopped clams, drained, juices reserved

    ½ cup fat-free half-and-half

    ¼ teaspoon red pepper flakes

    ¼ cup chopped fresh parsley

    2 tablespoons fresh lemon juice

    1 ounce freshly grated Parmesan cheese (¼ cup)

Cook pasta according to package directions. Drain and set aside.

While pasta is cooking, heat oil in a large skillet over medium heat. Add garlic and cook, stirring constantly, until fragrant, 30 seconds.

Add clam juice, half-and-half, and red pepper flakes; increase heat to high, bring to a boil, and cook until sauce is reduced and slightly thickened, about 10 minutes. Add parsley, lemon juice, clams, and pasta and toss until well combined. Sprinkle with Parmesan and serve.

Makes 4 (1¼-cup) servings

NUTRITION AT A GLANCE

Per serving: 340 calories, 7 g fat, 2 g saturated fat, 22 g protein, 50 g carbohydrate, 7 g dietary fiber, 1,060 mg sodium

Crab and Avocado Salad

PREP TIME: 10 minutes

This delectable multi-use recipe makes a great entrée salad or an appetizer in half-sized portions. In later phases, it can be an hors d'oeuvre on whole-grain crackers or a sandwich or wrap filling. Serve it as is or with a simple mixed green salad. If crabmeat is unavailable, cold steamed shrimp is just as good.

¼ cup chopped fresh cilantro

2 tablespoons mayonnaise

1 tablespoon chopped roasted red pepper (from a jar)

1 tablespoon fresh lime juice

⅛ teaspoon cayenne pepper

1 pound lump crabmeat

1 large ripe avocado, pitted, peeled, and cut into ¼-inch cubes

Salt and freshly ground black pepper

Combine cilantro, mayonnaise, red pepper, lime juice, and cayenne in a medium mixing bowl. Mix in crabmeat and season with salt and pepper. Gently fold in avocado and serve.

Makes 4 (scant 1-cup) servings

NUTRITION AT A GLANCE

Per serving: 230 calories, 14 g fat, 2 g saturated fat, 22 g protein, 4 g carbohydrate, 3 g dietary fiber, 670 mg sodium

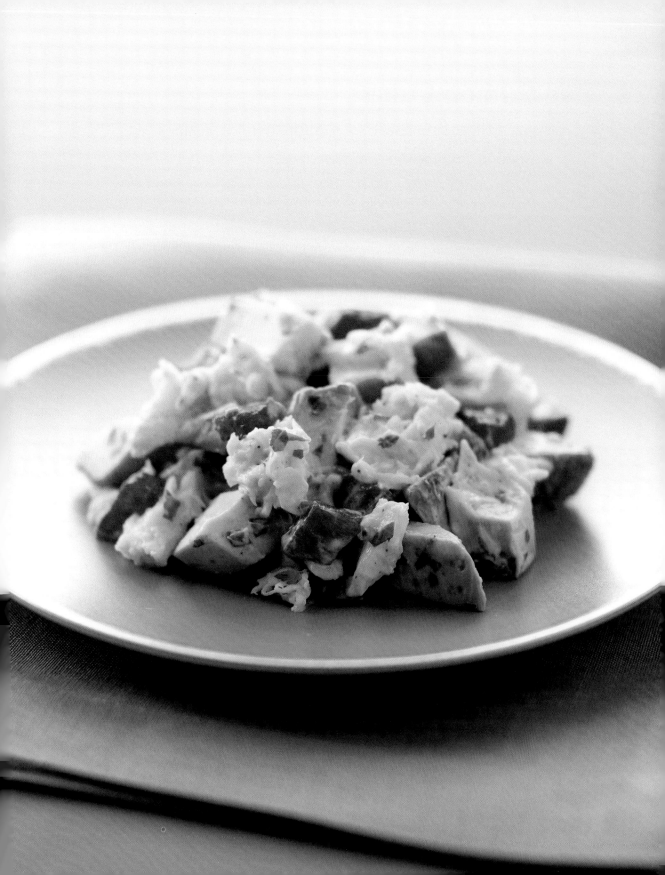

Salmon Cakes

PREP TIME: 10 minutes   **COOK TIME:** 12 minutes

These luscious cakes brim with the flavors of lemon and thyme. Serve them with a fresh salad or a favorite grain dish in Phases 2 and 3. If you don't have leftover cooked salmon, simply season a 1½-pound fillet with salt and pepper, place in a large skillet, add water just to cover, and poach until cooked through, about 8 to 10 minutes. Discard the skin, chop up the fish, and cool for 10 minutes before proceeding with the recipe.

> 1 large egg, lightly beaten
>
> ½ small red onion, minced
>
> 1 tablespoon fresh lemon juice
>
> 1½ teaspoons dried thyme
>
> 1½ teaspoons Dijon mustard
>
> 4 cups loosely packed chopped cooked salmon
>
> 1 teaspoon extra-virgin olive oil
>
> ¼ cup reduced-fat sour cream
>
> Salt and freshly ground black pepper

Whisk together egg, onion, lemon juice, thyme, mustard, ¾ teaspoon salt, and ¼ teaspoon pepper in a large mixing bowl. Add salmon and gently stir together. Form into 4 patties, about ¾ inch thick (cakes can be prepared up to 1 day ahead; wrap separately and refrigerate).

Heat oil over medium heat in a large cast-iron or nonstick skillet. Reduce heat to medium-low, lower salmon cakes into pan with a spatula, and cook until browned, cooking in batches if necessary, 5 minutes per side (because the cakes do not have bread crumbs, they may appear liquidy before they enter the pan). Serve warm with sour cream.

Makes 4 servings

NUTRITION AT A GLANCE

Per serving: 350 calories, 22 g fat, 5 g saturated fat, 34 g protein, 3 g carbohydrate, 0 g dietary fiber, 230 mg sodium

Baked Catfish with Lemon Aioli

PREP TIME: 5 minutes   **COOK TIME: 14 minutes**

Aioli—a fancy term for garlic-flavored mayonnaise—can be easily made at home with store-bought mayo. It makes a great sauce for this and other fish dishes.

  1 teaspoon dried thyme

  ⅛ teaspoon cayenne pepper

1½ pounds catfish fillets

  ¼ cup mayonnaise

1½ teaspoons fresh lemon juice

  1 small garlic clove, minced

    Salt and freshly ground black pepper

Heat oven to 400°F. Mix together thyme and cayenne and rub onto catfish; season fish on both sides with salt and pepper.

Lightly coat a 9- by 13-inch baking dish with cooking spray. Bake fish until opaque and cooked throughout, about 14 minutes.

While fish is baking, combine mayonnaise, lemon juice, and garlic in a small mixing bowl to make aioli. Serve fish hot with aioli.

Makes 4 servings

NUTRITION AT A GLANCE

Per serving: 330 calories, 24 g fat, 4.5 g saturated fat, 27 g protein, 1 g carbohydrate, 0 g dietary fiber, 250 mg sodium

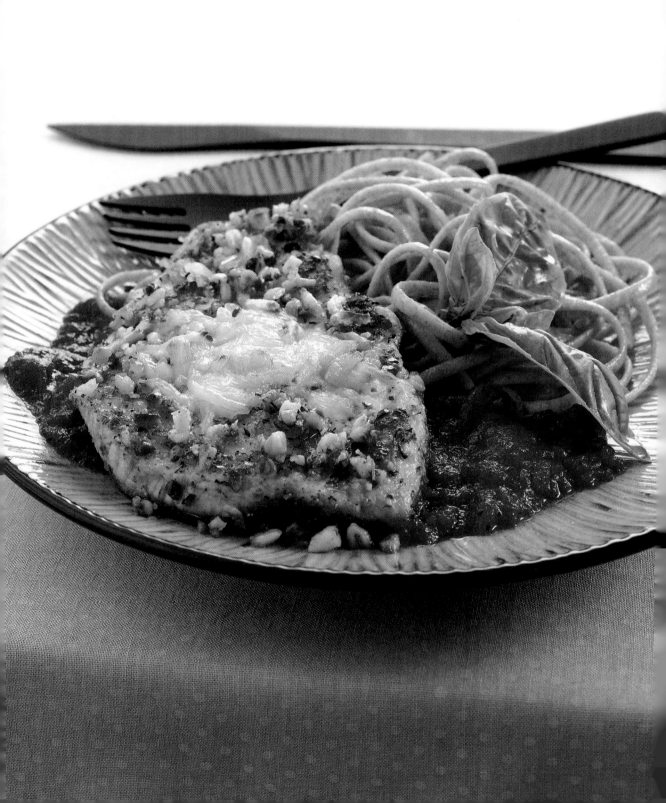

POULTRY

Hot, cold, in salads and stews, on skewers, in curries, or with whole-wheat pasta or couscous—you'll be amazed when you see how many healthful ways you can swiftly prepare skinless chicken and turkey. If available, try free-range poultry, which often has a better flavor.

In this chapter we introduce a host of exciting quick sauces, like Piri Piri—a spicy Portuguese and African condiment made with vinegar, garlic, and jalapeño peppers. Recipes like Chicken Breasts Stuffed with Spinach and Goat Cheese liven up a midweek meal, and Chicken Pot Pie and Turkey Noodle Soup are perfect for chilly days when a little dose of comfort fits the bill.

A few good spices, such as cajun seasoning, and store-bought condiments, such as green curry paste, will help you cut prep time while keeping flavor top of mind. Or try our quick barbecue sauce for a juicy, tangy, baked barbecue chicken any night of the year.

◄ *Turkey Parmesan (page 252)*

Turkey Parmesan

PREP TIME: 10 minutes   **COOK TIME:** 15 minutes

We love this version of the Italian classic. Pine nuts replace the usual flour coating, adding crunchy texture and nutty flavor. Serve with whole-wheat pasta for a Phase 2 dinner your whole family will love. If you don't have Italian seasoning on hand, use dried basil, rosemary, or thyme— or a mix of all three!

    2 cups low-sugar pasta sauce

    ½ cup pine nuts, coarsely chopped

    1 ounce freshly grated Parmesan cheese (¼ cup)

    ½ teaspoon dried Italian seasoning

    1 pound turkey cutlets, about ⅓ inch thick

    2 teaspoons extra-virgin olive oil

    2 ounces shredded part-skim mozzarella cheese (½ cup)

    Salt and freshly ground black pepper

Heat oven to broil. Bring sauce to low simmer in a small saucepan over medium-low heat. Remove from heat and cover to keep warm.

Stir together pine nuts, Parmesan, and Italian seasoning in a wide, shallow dish. Season turkey on both sides with salt and pepper, then dredge both sides in the nut mixture, pressing to adhere.

Heat oil in a large nonstick skillet over medium-low heat. Add turkey and cook until coating is golden brown and juices run clear, about 4 minutes per side. If nuts brown too quickly, reduce heat.

Place turkey in a baking pan, top evenly with mozzarella, and broil until cheese melts, about 30 seconds.

Spoon ½ cup of warm sauce on each plate and top each with a piece of turkey.

Makes 4 servings

NUTRITION AT A GLANCE

Per serving: 380 calories, 21 g fat, 4 g saturated fat, 39 g protein, 10 g carbohydrate, 3 g dietary fiber, 650 mg sodium

Indian Chicken

PREP TIME: 10 minutes   **COOK TIME: 20 minutes**

Coconut milk, curry powder, garlic, and ginger create a warmly spiced, full-bodied broth. Add tender chicken and sweet cauliflower and you've got a surprisingly easy, sumptuous one-pan dish.

1½ pounds boneless, skinless chicken breasts, cut into 1-inch pieces

1 tablespoon canola oil

1 small onion, diced

2 garlic cloves, minced

1 tablespoon curry powder

1 teaspoon ground ginger

1 (2-pound) head cauliflower, cut into florets (4 cups)

1 (13.5-ounce) can light coconut milk

½ cup lower-sodium chicken broth or water

Salt and freshly ground black pepper

Season chicken well with salt and pepper. Heat oil in a large skillet over medium-high heat; add chicken and cook until lightly browned, about 5 minutes. Using a slotted spoon, transfer chicken to a plate.

Reduce heat to medium-low. Add onion, garlic, curry powder, and ginger to the same skillet. Cook until fragrant, about 2 minutes. Add cauliflower, coconut milk, and broth; cover and simmer, stirring occasionally, until vegetables are crisp-tender, about 5 minutes. Add chicken back to the pan and cook until sauce is thickened and reduced, about 5 minutes. Serve hot.

Makes 4 (2-cup) servings

NUTRITION AT A GLANCE

Per serving: 340 calories, 13 g fat, 6 g saturated fat, 44 g protein, 12 g carbohydrate, 3 g dietary fiber, 250 mg sodium

Rigatoni with Turkey Sausage and Mozzarella

PREP TIME: 5 minutes   **COOK TIME: 20 minutes**

You can use sweet or hot Italian turkey sausage for this dish—either one blends perfectly with the pasta sauce and fresh basil.

8 ounces spelt or whole-wheat rigatoni or penne

¾ pound reduced-fat sweet or hot Italian turkey sausages

3 cups low-sugar pasta sauce

4 ounces shredded part-skim mozzarella cheese (1 cup)

½ cup chopped fresh basil

Salt and freshly ground black pepper

Cook pasta according to package directions. Drain and set aside.

While pasta is cooking, heat a large nonstick skillet over medium heat. Add sausages and cook, turning often, until no longer pink inside, about 15 minutes. Transfer to a cutting board and slice diagonally into ¼-inch-thick pieces.

Heat pasta sauce over medium heat until hot. Place pasta, sausage, sauce, cheese, and basil in a large bowl and toss to combine. Season with salt and pepper and serve hot.

Makes 4 (2-cup) servings

NUTRITION AT A GLANCE

Per serving: 460 calories, 16 g fat, 5 g saturated fat, 33 g protein, 42 g carbohydrate, 10 g dietary fiber, 1,030 mg sodium

Chicken Jambalaya

PREP TIME: 10 minutes   **COOK TIME:** 35 minutes

A classic Louisiana dish, jambalaya can be made with any combination of beef, pork, chicken, sausage, ham, or seafood; feel free to use a mixture of proteins, if you'd like. This recipe cooks in just over 30 minutes, but it's worth the extra time especially if you're having friends over for dinner. Heat lovers: Add more Cajun seasoning or cayenne.

1½ pounds boneless, skinless chicken breasts, cut into bite-size pieces

2 tablespoons extra-virgin olive oil, divided

2 bunches scallions, white and green parts, chopped (2 tablespoons reserved for garnish)

1 green bell pepper, chopped

2 garlic cloves, minced

½ cup whole-grain, quick-cooking brown rice (page 14)

⅛ teaspoon sugar-free Cajun seasoning or cayenne pepper

2 cups lower-sodium chicken broth

1 (14-ounce) can diced tomatoes

Salt and freshly ground black pepper

Season chicken with salt and pepper. Heat 1 tablespoon of the oil in a large straight-sided skillet over medium-high heat. Add chicken, scallions, bell pepper, and garlic; cook, stirring often, until vegetables are softened, about 5 minutes.

Stir in rice and Cajun seasoning. Add broth and tomatoes with juice and bring to a boil. Reduce heat to medium-low, cover, and simmer, stirring occasionally, until most of the liquid is absorbed, about 30 minutes. If jambalaya has excess moisture, cook uncovered for 3 to 5 minutes. Sprinkle with reserved scallions and serve.

Makes 4 (1½-cup) servings

NUTRITION AT A GLANCE

Per serving: 400 calories, 11 g fat, 2 g saturated fat, 46 g protein, 29 g carbohydrate, 4 g dietary fiber, 550 mg sodium

Ginger Chicken with Snow Pea Salad

PREP TIME: 10 minutes   **COOK TIME:** 20 minutes

Ginger lovers will fall hard for this easy chicken dish, which can be topped with sesame seeds for extra pizzazz.

  1 pound snow peas, strings removed

  1 tablespoon plus 2 teaspoons canola oil, divided

  1 tablespoon plus 1 teaspoon low-sodium soy sauce, divided

  1 tablespoon minced fresh ginger

1½ pounds boneless, skinless chicken breasts

  2 scallions, sliced

  2 teaspoons dark sesame oil

Bring a medium saucepan of salted water to a boil. Fill a medium mixing bowl with ice and water. Boil snow peas for 2 minutes, drain, and place in ice water for 1 minute to chill. Drain and pat dry.

Combine 2 teaspoons of the canola oil, 1 tablespoon of the soy sauce, and ginger in a shallow bowl. Add chicken and toss to coat.

Heat remaining canola oil in a large skillet over medium-high heat. Add chicken and cook until golden and no longer pink inside, 5 minutes per side. Transfer to a cutting board and slice.

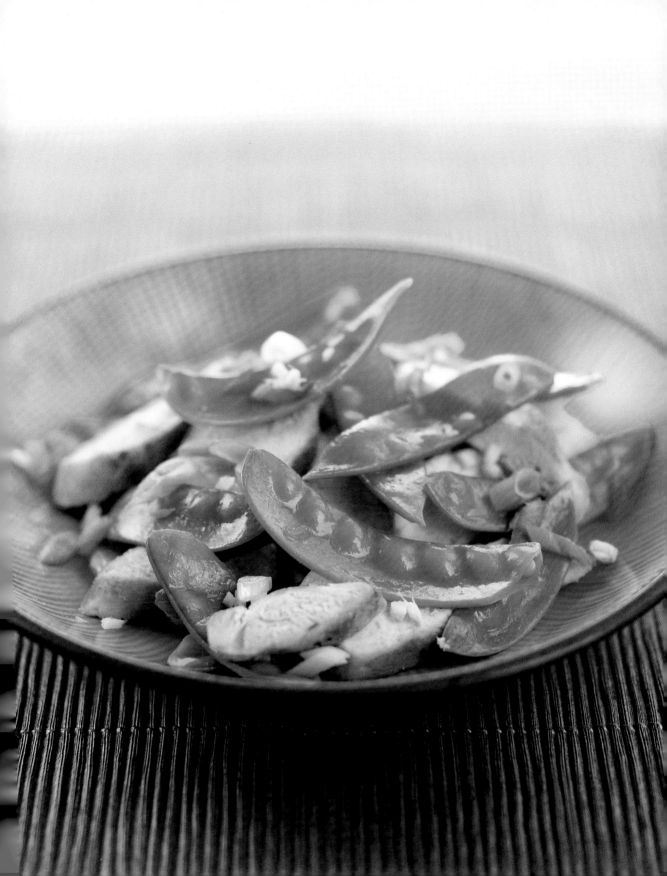

Combine peas, scallions, sesame oil, and remaining soy sauce in a mixing bowl; toss together. Serve pea salad with chicken.

Makes 4 servings

NUTRITION AT A GLANCE

Per serving: 310 calories, 11 g fat, 1.5 g saturated fat, 43 g protein, 10 g carbohydrate, 2 g dietary fiber, 320 mg sodium

Chinese-Style Steamed Chicken

PREP TIME: 15 minutes   **COOK TIME:** 15 minutes

Using packaged broccoli florets and jarred minced garlic will help you cut the prep time for this recipe. If you have extra time, let the chicken marinate in the soy sauce mixture for 30 minutes for added flavor.

- 4 (6-ounce) boneless, skinless chicken breasts
- 4 garlic cloves, minced
- 1 teaspoon minced fresh ginger
- 4 scallions, chopped
- 2 tablespoons low-sodium soy sauce
- 1 teaspoon red pepper flakes
- 1 (1-pound) head broccoli, cut into florets (3½ to 4 cups)

Fill bottom part of a steamer with 1 inch of water; bring to boil.

Toss chicken with garlic, ginger, scallions, soy sauce, and red pepper flakes, coating breasts well. Place chicken in the steamer basket, pouring remaining soy sauce mixture over chicken. Lower basket into water container, reduce to a rapid simmer, and cover with a lid. Steam for 5 minutes.

Turn chicken breasts, add broccoli, cover, and

continue steaming until chicken is cooked through and broccoli is tender, 5 to 6 minutes more. Serve hot.

Makes 4 servings

NUTRITION AT A GLANCE

Per serving: 220 calories, 2.5 g fat, ½ g saturated fat, 42 g protein, 6 g carbohydrate, 2 g dietary fiber, 430 mg sodium

Chicken Quesadillas

PREP TIME: 5 minutes   **COOK TIME: 15 minutes**

Melted cheese over tender chicken and creamy avocado couldn't be better—unless of course it's topped with juicy tomato salsa, as it is here. These quesadillas cook up fast for lunch or dinner.

4 (8-inch) whole-wheat tortillas

1 cup shredded reduced-fat cheddar or Jack cheese

2 (6-ounce) boneless, skinless chicken breasts, cooked and cut into ½-inch slices

1 avocado, pitted, peeled, and thinly sliced

2 scallions, thinly sliced

½ cup refrigerated fresh salsa

Salt and freshly ground black pepper

Heat oven to 200°F.

Heat 1 tortilla in a large nonstick skillet (wider than the tortilla) over medium heat until warm, about 1 minute. Sprinkle with one-quarter each of the cheese, chicken, avocado, and scallions and a pinch of salt and pepper.

Cover and cook until the cheese is melted, about 2 minutes. Transfer to a cutting board, fold the tortilla in half, and place on a baking sheet in the oven to keep warm. Repeat to use remaining ingredients. Cut each quesadilla into 3 triangles and serve with salsa.

Makes 4 servings

NUTRITION AT A GLANCE

Per serving: 370 calories, 13 g fat, 2.5 g saturated fat, 32 g protein, 29 g carbohydrate, 5 g dietary fiber, 580 mg sodium

Provolone Chicken Melts

PREP TIME: 5 minutes   **COOK TIME: 15 minutes**

These cheesy open-faced sandwiches are so gooey you'll want to eat them with a knife and fork. You can use grilled, baked, or poached chicken instead of pan cooked, if you prefer.

- 4 (6-ounce) boneless, skinless chicken breasts
- 4 teaspoons extra-virgin olive oil, divided
- 4 slices multigrain bread
- 1 large garlic clove, cut in half
- 1 whole roasted bell pepper (from a jar), cut into 4 pieces
- 4 (¾-ounce) slices reduced-fat provolone or Monterey Jack cheese

  Salt and freshly ground black pepper

Heat oven to broil.

Lightly pound each chicken breast to an even thickness and season with salt and pepper. Heat 2 teaspoons of the oil in a large nonstick skillet over medium heat. Sauté chicken until cooked through, about 5 minutes per side. Transfer to a plate.

Lay bread slices on a baking sheet, drizzle with remaining oil, and rub with the cut sides of the garlic clove; discard garlic. Place under the broiler until toasted, about 1 minute.

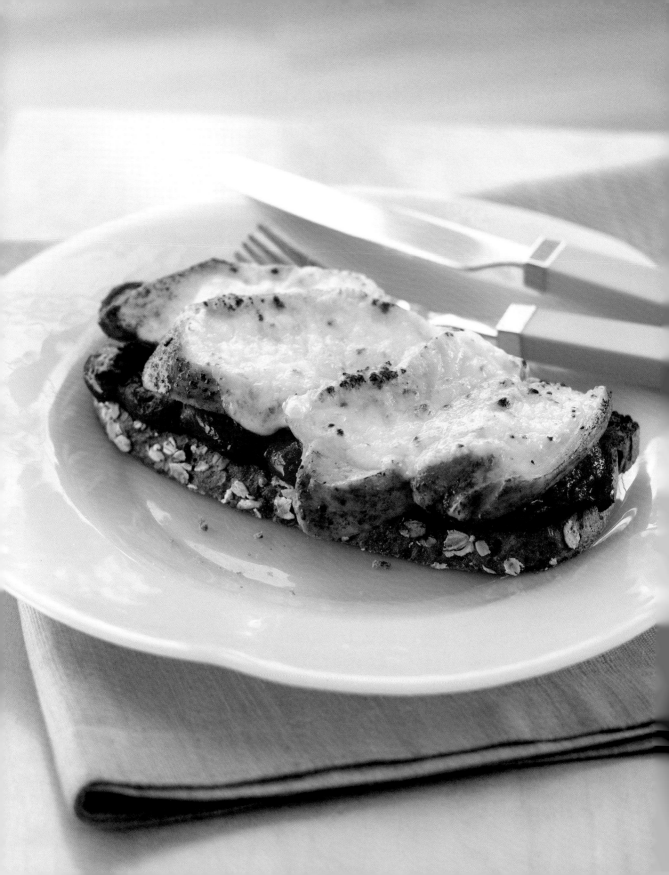

Top each bread slice with 1 pepper piece, 1 chicken breast, and 1 cheese slice. Broil until cheese has melted, about 2 minutes. Serve hot.

Makes 4 servings

NUTRITION AT A GLANCE

Per serving: 350 calories, 12 g fat, 3.5 g saturated fat, 49 g protein, 13 g carbohydrate, 2 g dietary fiber, 340 mg sodium

Tomato-Saffron Stewed Chicken

PREP TIME: 10 minutes   **COOK TIME:** 30 minutes

Saffron's flavor and exquisite color bring something special to this quick and simple stew. The spice is more expensive than most others, but the good news is that a little goes a long way. Store it in a cool, dark pantry so it keeps well and you can enjoy it for many months.

- 4 (6-ounce) boneless, skinless chicken breasts, cut in half crosswise on the diagonal
- 2 tablespoons extra-virgin olive oil
- 1 medium onion, thinly sliced
- 2 garlic cloves, minced
- 1 (28-ounce) can unsalted diced tomatoes
- ¼ teaspoon powdered saffron
- ¼ cup fresh parsley leaves, roughly chopped
- Salt and freshly ground black pepper

Season chicken with salt and pepper. Heat oil in a large, heavy-bottomed saucepan over medium-high heat. Add chicken and cook until chicken is lightly browned, 3 minutes per side. Remove chicken from pan.

Add onion and garlic to the same skillet and cook over medium-high heat for 2 minutes. Return chicken to pan, add tomatoes with juice and saffron, bring to a low boil, reduce to a simmer, and cook until sauce has thickened and chicken is cooked through, about 15 minutes. Stir in parsley, season with salt and pepper, and serve.

Makes 4 servings

NUTRITION AT A GLANCE

Per serving: 300 calories, 9 g fat, 1.5 g saturated fat, 41 g protein, 13 g carbohydrate, 4 g dietary fiber, 190 mg sodium

Turkey Sausages with Kale and Chickpeas

PREP TIME: 10 minutes   **COOK TIME:** 30 minutes

Chock-full of vitamins A and C, folic acid, calcium, and iron, kale plays a key role in this easy protein- and fiber-rich dish. Look for turkey sausage free from nitrates, sugars, and fillers, such as bread (page 13).

- 1 tablespoon extra-virgin olive oil
- 1 pound reduced-fat sweet or hot Italian turkey sausages
- 1 small onion, diced
- 3 garlic cloves, minced
- 1½ cups lower-sodium chicken broth
- 1 (1-pound) bunch kale, stemmed and roughly chopped (6 to 7 cups)
- 1 (15-ounce) can chickpeas, rinsed and drained
- Salt and freshly ground black pepper

Heat oil in a large saucepan over medium-high heat. Add sausages and cook until browned on all sides, turning occasionally, 6 minutes. Remove from pan and cut each sausage in half on the diagonal.

Add onion and garlic to the same saucepan and cook over medium heat until softened and translucent, about 3 minutes. Add broth and bring to a simmer. Add kale, cover, and cook until wilted and softened, about 8 minutes.

Add sausages and cook, covered, until no longer pink in the center, about 8 minutes. Add chickpeas and continue cooking, covered, until heated through, 2 minutes. Season to taste with salt and pepper and serve hot, spooning any remaining cooking liquid on top.

Makes 4 (1½-cup) servings

NUTRITION AT A GLANCE

Per serving: 340 calories, 11 g fat, 2.5 g saturated fat, 31 g protein, 32 g carbohydrate, 6 g dietary fiber, 1,090 mg sodium

Chicken Piri-Piri

PREP TIME: 20 minutes (includes marinating)
COOK TIME: 10 minutes

This deliciously spicy chicken dish has both Portuguese and African origins. We've taken a touch of the heat out by removing the jalapeño seeds from the chili marinade, but you can amp it up by leaving them in, if you dare!

¼ cup extra-virgin olive oil

2 tablespoons cider vinegar

1 jalapeño pepper, seeded and minced

1 garlic clove, minced

¼ teaspoon red pepper flakes

¼ teaspoon salt

4 (6-ounce) boneless, skinless chicken breasts

Heat grill or grill pan to high.

Whisk together oil, vinegar, jalapeño, garlic, red pepper flakes, and salt in a small bowl. Place chicken in a shallow dish. Add 3 tablespoons of the marinade and turn to coat. Let stand at room temperature 10 minutes.

Grill chicken, turning often, until juices run clear, about 10 minutes. Drizzle with remaining sauce (do not use any of the leftover marinade) and serve.

Makes 4 servings

NUTRITION AT A GLANCE

Per serving: 310 calories, 16 g fat, 2.5 g saturated fat, 39 g protein, 1 g carbohydrate, 0 g dietary fiber, 260 mg sodium

Grilled Chicken with Garlic, Olive, and Tomato Salsa

PREP TIME: 10 minutes   **COOK TIME:** 10 minutes

A simple mix of classic Mediterranean ingredients turns chicken into a delicious savory dish that's perfect weeknight fare. Try a mixed variety of olives, if you'd like, and remember that olives are naturally salty so use a light hand when seasoning the salsa.

1 cup pitted kalamata olives, chopped

1 plum tomato, seeded and diced

1 garlic clove, minced

1 teaspoon red wine vinegar

½ teaspoon dried oregano

2 tablespoons extra-virgin olive oil, divided

¼ cup fresh parsley leaves (optional)

4 (6-ounce) boneless, skinless chicken breasts

Salt and freshly ground black pepper

Combine olives, tomato, garlic, vinegar, oregano, and 1 tablespoon of the oil in a mixing bowl. Toss with parsley, if using, and season to taste with salt and pepper.

Heat grill or grill pan to medium-high. Rub chicken with remaining oil and season with salt and pepper. Grill until no longer pink inside, about 4 minutes per side. Serve warm with salsa.

Makes 4 servings

NUTRITION AT A GLANCE

Per serving: 330 calories, 17 g fat, 2.5 g saturated fat, 40 g protein, 4 g carbohydrate, 0 g dietary fiber, 570 mg sodium

Chicken Breasts Stuffed with Spinach and Goat Cheese

PREP TIME: 15 minutes   COOK TIME: 15 minutes

This creamy, garlic-filled chicken is perfect for entertaining. Stuff the chicken ahead of time and dinner will cook up in minutes. If you don't have an ovenproof skillet (one with a heatproof handle made from stainless steel, cast iron, or aluminum), transfer the chicken to a baking dish before baking. When removing an ovenproof skillet from the oven, remember that the handle is extremely hot. Be sure to use a thick pot holder and leave it over the handle once the pan is removed from the oven so that others know not to touch.

4 teaspoons extra-virgin olive oil, divided

2 garlic cloves, minced

1 (½-pound) bunch spinach, tough stems removed

4 (6-ounce) boneless, skinless chicken breasts

4 ounces low-fat goat cheese

   Salt and freshly ground black pepper

Special equipment:

   Wooden toothpicks

Heat oven to 400°F.

   Heat 2 teaspoons of the oil in a large ovenproof skillet over medium heat. Add garlic and cook, stirring constantly, until fragrant, about 30 seconds. Stir in spinach and cook, stirring constantly, until spinach is wilted and liquid evaporates, about 2 minutes. Season well with salt and pepper and transfer to a plate. Wipe skillet dry with paper towels.

Beginning at the thickest end of 1 chicken breast, carefully insert a sharp knife into center and cut a pocket as evenly as possible, leaving a 1-inch border on three sides. Repeat with remaining breasts. Open each pocket, sprinkle with salt and pepper, then fill evenly with goat cheese and spinach. Seal each with two toothpicks and season outside with salt and pepper.

Heat remaining oil in the same skillet over medium-high heat. Add chicken and cook, turning once, until well browned on both sides, about 3 minutes per side. Transfer the skillet to the oven and bake until juices run clear, about 8 minutes. Serve hot.

Makes 4 servings

NUTRITION AT A GLANCE

Per serving: 280 calories, 10 g fat, 3 g saturated fat, 42 g protein, 3 g carbohydrate, 1 g dietary fiber, 390 mg sodium

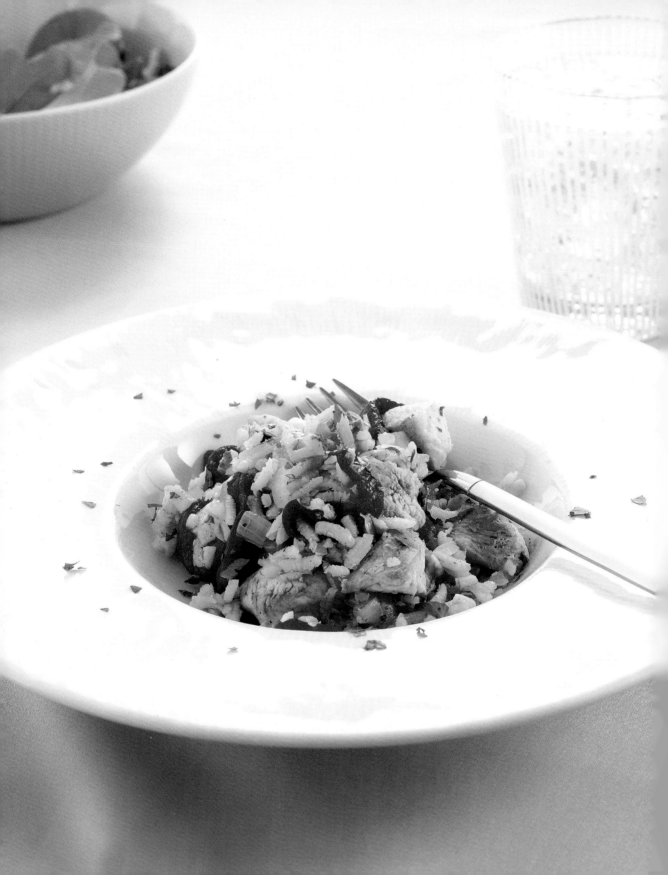

South Beach Chicken Paella

PREP TIME: 10 minutes   **COOK TIME: 35 minutes**

Saffron makes this simple one-pan classic a real treat, lending brilliant color and pungent flavor. This is one of the few recipes that takes a little bit longer to cook than most of the others in this book; it's a great dish to serve for company.

- 1½ pounds boneless, skinless chicken breasts, cut into ½-inch pieces
- 1 tablespoon extra-virgin olive oil
- 1 medium onion, chopped
- ½ cup whole-grain, quick-cooking brown rice (page 14)
- ¾ cup roasted red bell peppers (from a jar), drained and thinly sliced
- 2 cups lower-sodium chicken broth
- ¼ teaspoon powdered saffron
- 3 tablespoons chopped fresh parsley

  Salt and freshly ground black pepper

Season chicken with salt and pepper. Heat oil in a large, straight-sided skillet over medium-high heat. Add chicken and onion; cook, stirring often, until onion is softened, about 5 minutes.

Stir in rice. Add red peppers, broth, and saffron; bring to a boil. Cover, reduce heat, and simmer, stirring occasionally, until most of the liquid is absorbed, about 30 minutes. If paella has excess moisture, cook uncovered for 3 to 5 minutes. Stir in parsley, season to taste with salt and pepper, and serve.

Makes 4 (1½-cup) servings

NUTRITION AT A GLANCE

Per serving: 360 calories, 7 g fat, 1.5 g saturated fat, 45 g protein, 26 g carbohydrate, 1 g dietary fiber, 440 mg sodium

Turkey Swedish Meatballs

PREP TIME: 10 minutes   **COOK TIME:** 15 minutes

These spiced meatballs are breadless. Though you'll find them to be moister than traditional meatballs when forming, they cook up just the same way and are just as delicious. Still, as the old advice goes, be careful not to overmix. Serve with a salad or in later phases over whole-wheat pasta.

¾ teaspoon salt

½ teaspoon ground allspice

¼ teaspoon freshly ground black pepper

1 pound ground turkey breast

1 tablespoon extra-virgin olive oil

¾ cup lower-sodium chicken broth

3 tablespoons reduced-fat sour cream

2 tablespoons chopped fresh parsley

Mix together salt, allspice, and pepper in a medium mixing bowl. Add turkey and gently mix with hands to combine; shape into 24 (1-inch) balls.

Heat oil in a large nonstick skillet over medium-high heat. Add meatballs and cook until browned, about 3 minutes; lower heat to medium and cook 3 more minutes, gently shaking pan. Using a slotted spoon, transfer meatballs to a plate.

Add broth to the same skillet, increase heat to medium-high, and simmer until liquid is reduced by half, about 5 minutes. Whisk in sour cream and cook 1 minute more. Add meatballs. Sprinkle with parsley and serve hot.

Makes 4 servings

NUTRITION AT A GLANCE

Per serving: 180 calories, 7 g fat, 1.5 g saturated fat, 29 g protein, 1 g carbohydrate, 0 g dietary fiber, 230 mg sodium

Peanut Chicken with Noodles

PREP TIME: 15 minutes   **COOK TIME: 20 minutes**

Creamy peanut butter, dark sesame oil, and Japanese soba noodles give this dish a punch of protein and delicious nutty flavor. If you don't want to fire up the grill, simply poach, bake, or pan-cook the chicken. Look for soba noodles and rice vinegar in the Asian section of your supermarket or health food store.

- 4 ounces soba noodles
- 1½ pounds boneless, skinless chicken breasts
- 3 teaspoons dark sesame oil, divided
- ⅓ cup creamy trans-fat-free peanut butter
- 2 tablespoons low-sodium soy sauce
- 2 tablespoons rice vinegar
- 2 tablespoons water
- 1 (¾-pound) head napa cabbage, shredded (4 cups)
- 2 scallions, thinly sliced
- Salt and freshly ground black pepper

Cook noodles according to package directions; run under cool water and drain.

Season chicken well with salt and pepper and toss with 1 teaspoon of the oil. Heat grill pan or skillet over medium-high heat; cook chicken until browned and cooked through, about 4 minutes per side. Transfer to a cutting board.

Whisk together peanut butter, soy sauce, vinegar, water, and remaining oil in a large mixing bowl. Thinly slice chicken and add to peanut butter mixture. Add noodles, cabbage, and scallions; toss gently to combine and serve.

Makes 4 (2-cup) servings

NUTRITION AT A GLANCE

Per serving: 370 calories, 13 g fat, 2.5 g saturated fat, 42 g protein, 19 g carbohydrate, 2 g dietary fiber, 500 mg sodium

Chicken Couscous

PREP TIME: 15 minutes   **COOK TIME:** 10 minutes

Put a few pantry staples together and you'll have this deliciously spiced, authentic-style couscous on the table lickety-split.

 1 pound boneless, skinless chicken breasts, cut into ¾-inch cubes

 1 tablespoon extra-virgin olive oil

 1 small onion, diced

 ½ teaspoon ground cumin

 ¼ teaspoon ground cinnamon

 1 cup lower-sodium chicken broth

 ½ cup whole-wheat couscous

 1 (15-ounce) can chickpeas, rinsed and drained

    Salt and freshly ground black pepper

Season chicken with salt and pepper. Heat oil in a large saucepan over medium-high heat. Cook chicken until no longer pink inside and lightly browned, about 6 minutes. Remove chicken from pan with a slotted spoon and drain on paper towels.

Reduce heat to medium and add onion, cumin, and cinnamon to the same pan; cook until onions are softened and lightly browned, about 3 minutes. Add broth and bring to a simmer. Stir in couscous, chickpeas, and a good pinch of salt and pepper. Reduce heat to low, cover, and cook 1 minute. Return chicken to saucepan, combine with couscous, season to taste with salt and pepper, and serve.

Makes 4 (1½-cup) servings

NUTRITION AT A GLANCE

Per serving: 320 calories, 6 g fat, 1 g saturated fat, 33 g protein, 32 g carbohydrate, 6 g dietary fiber, 400 mg sodium

Curried Chicken Salad

PREP TIME: 15 minutes

Serve this sensational salad as is or try it inside half of a large scooped-out tomato or on top of fresh salad greens. In later phases, use it as a sandwich filling inside a whole-wheat pita.

1½ cups plain fat-free or low-fat yogurt

1 tablespoon curry powder

½ teaspoon ground ginger

1½ pounds boneless, skinless chicken breasts, cooked and cut into ½-inch cubes

3 celery stalks, diced

½ small red onion, diced

¼ cup chopped fresh cilantro

Salt and freshly ground black pepper

Whisk together yogurt, curry powder, and ginger in a large mixing bowl. Stir in chicken, celery, onion, and cilantro; season to taste with salt and pepper. Serve at room temperature or refrigerate for at least 1 hour before serving for more concentrated flavor.

Makes 4 (1-cup) servings

NUTRITION AT A GLANCE

Per serving: 240 calories, 2.5 g fat, .5 g saturated fat, 44 g protein, 11 g carbohydrate, 1 g dietary fiber, 270 mg sodium

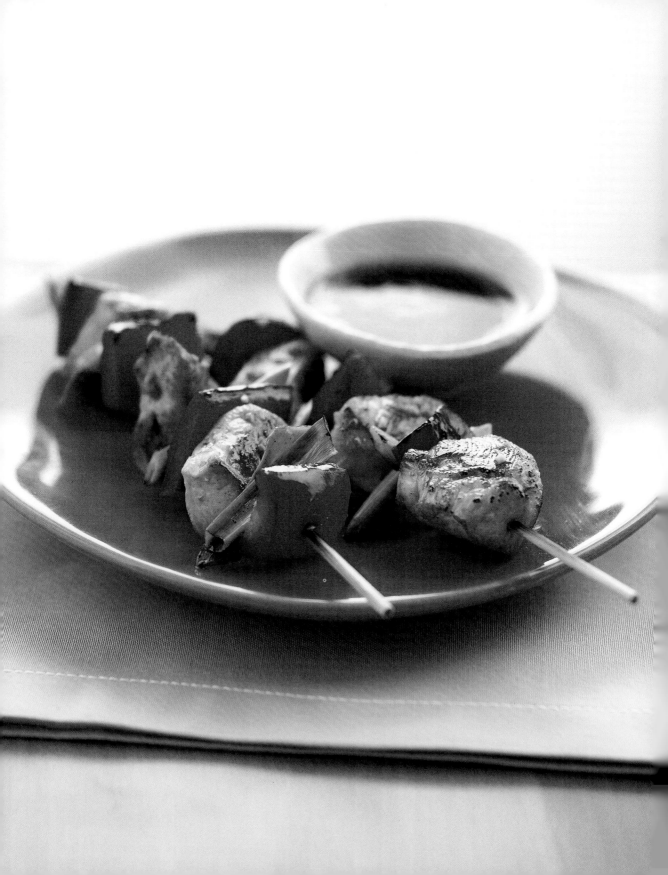

Chicken Yakitori

PREP TIME: 10 minutes
COOK TIME: 20 minutes (includes marinating)

Sprightly ginger and sesame flavors coat these tender skewers, which make for fun fare any night of the week. In later phases, serve them with Nutty Brown Rice (page 421). Look for mirin or rice wine in the Asian section of your supermarket or health food store or simply substitute ⅓ cup dry white wine plus 2 teaspoons granular sugar substitute.

1½ pounds boneless, skinless chicken breasts, cut into 1-inch pieces

10 scallions, cut into 1-inch pieces

1 large red bell pepper, cut into 1-inch squares

⅓ cup low-sodium soy sauce

3 tablespoons mirin or rice wine (page 38)

2 teaspoons dark sesame oil

2 tablespoons grated fresh ginger

2 garlic cloves, minced

Special equipment:

8 (8-inch) skewers (if wooden, soak in water for 30 minutes)

Heat oven to broil.

Thread chicken, scallions, and pepper onto skewers; place in a large shallow dish. Whisk together soy sauce, mirin, oil, ginger, and garlic. Cover skewers with ½ cup

of the mixture and marinate at room temperature for
10 minutes; set aside remaining soy sauce mixture for
dressing cooked skewers.

Lightly coat a broiler pan with cooking spray. Place
skewers on the pan, reserving marinade. Broil, turning
skewers and basting occasionally with reserved
marinade, until chicken is no longer pink, about
10 minutes.

Serve hot with reserved soy sauce mixture.

Makes 4 servings

NUTRITION AT A GLANCE

Per serving: 270 calories, 4.5 g fat, 1 g saturated fat,
42 g protein, 12 g carbohydrate, 2 g dietary fiber,
830 mg sodium

Turkey and White Bean Chili

PREP TIME: 10 minutes   **COOK TIME:** 30 minutes

This yummy chili can be made many different ways, if you want to experiment. Try using chicken instead of turkey or navy, black, or pinto beans in place of the white ones. Top it with a tablespoon or two of shredded low-fat cheddar or jack cheese, sliced scallions, or chopped cilantro. You can even use chipotle chili powder for a smoky taste, in place of regular.

- 1 tablespoon extra-virgin olive oil
- 1 medium onion, roughly chopped
- 2 garlic cloves, minced
- 1 pound turkey cutlets, cut into ½-inch pieces
- 1 tablespoon chili powder
- 1 teaspoon ground cumin
- 1 (15-ounce) can cannellini beans, rinsed and drained
- 1 (14.5-ounce) can Mexican diced tomatoes
- 1 cup lower-sodium chicken broth
- Salt and freshly ground black pepper

Heat oil in a large saucepan over medium-high heat. Add onion and cook, stirring occasionally, until softened, about 5 minutes. Add garlic and cook 1 minute more.

Add turkey, chili powder, and cumin; cook, stirring often, until turkey is no longer pink inside, about 5 minutes.

Add beans, tomatoes with juice, and broth; bring to a boil. Reduce heat to medium-low, cover, and simmer until flavors blend, about 15 minutes. Season with salt and pepper to taste and serve.

Makes 4 (1¹⁄₄-cup) servings

NUTRITION AT A GLANCE

Per serving: 260 calories, 5 g fat, ¹⁄₂ g saturated fat, 34 g protein, 21 g carbohydrate, 6 g dietary fiber, 500 mg sodium

Baked Pesto Chicken

PREP TIME: 5 minutes   **COOK TIME:** 30 minutes

Store-bought pesto and mozzarella cheese are all it takes to turn tender chicken breasts into an incredibly easy-to-make dish that will likely become a new family favorite.

4 (6-ounce) boneless, skinless chicken breasts

½ cup pesto (from a jar)

2 ounces shredded part-skim mozzarella cheese (½ cup)

Salt and freshly ground black pepper

Heat oven to 375°F.

Season chicken with salt and pepper. Spread ¼ cup of the pesto in a 9- by 13-inch baking dish. Lay chicken breasts over pesto in an even layer and spread with remaining pesto.

Cover baking dish with foil and bake chicken until cooked through, 20 to 25 minutes. Uncover and top with cheese. Bake until cheese is melted, 5 more minutes. Serve hot.

Makes 4 servings

NUTRITION AT A GLANCE

Per serving: 390 calories, 20 g fat, 5 g saturated fat, 46 g protein, 2 g carbohydrate, 0 g dietary fiber, 450 mg sodium

Poached Chicken Sandwich with Lemon-Caper Mayo

PREP TIME: 10 minutes   **COOK TIME: 25 minutes**

Tender chicken breasts with a deliciously tangy dressing make a great sandwich that requires little cleanup. You can poach the chicken up to 2 days ahead; just remember to cool it completely before refrigerating.

- 4 cups water
- 1½ tablespoons fresh lemon juice, divided
- 4 (6-ounce) boneless, skinless chicken breasts
- ¼ cup mayonnaise
- 1 tablespoon capers, drained, rinsed, and roughly chopped
- 8 slices whole-grain bread, lightly toasted
- 4 lettuce leaves
- Salt and freshly ground black pepper

Bring water and 1 tablespoon of the lemon juice to a simmer in a large, high-sided saucepan. Season chicken with salt and pepper, add to water, and simmer, covered, 10 minutes. Remove pan from heat and let stand, covered, for 15 minutes. Remove to a plate and cool at room temperature, 5 minutes.

While chicken is cooking, mix together mayonnaise, remaining lemon juice, and capers. Season to taste with pepper.

Make each sandwich with 2 bread slices, 1 chicken breast (sliced in half lengthwise, if easier to manage), 2 tablespoons mayonnaise, and 1 lettuce leaf. Slice in half and serve.

Makes 4 servings

NUTRITION AT A GLANCE

Per serving: 420 calories, 15 g fat, 2.5 g saturated fat, 45 g protein, 25 g carbohydrate, 3 g dietary fiber, 540 mg sodium

Warm Kasha and Grilled Chicken Pilaf

PREP TIME: 10 minutes   **COOK TIME:** 10 minutes

Toasty, nutty kasha brings nutrition and great flavor to this delicious chicken salad. Try it for a picnic, take-along office lunch, or light dinner. Add chopped parsley for extra flavor and color if you have some on hand.

- ½ cup kasha
- 1¼ pounds boneless, skinless chicken breasts
- 3 tablespoons extra-virgin olive oil, divided
- 1 medium cucumber, peeled, seeded, and chopped
- ¼ cup finely chopped red onion
- 3 tablespoons fresh lemon juice
- Salt and freshly ground black pepper

Cook kasha according to package directions.

While kasha is cooking, heat grill or grill pan to medium-high. Toss chicken with 1 tablespoon of the oil, season with salt and pepper, and grill 4 to 5 minutes per side. Transfer chicken to a cutting board and allow to rest a few minutes, then slice into thin strips.

Toss chicken strips with cooked kasha, cucumber, onion, lemon juice, and remaining oil. Season with salt and pepper and serve warm.

Makes 4 (2-cup) servings

NUTRITION AT A GLANCE

Per serving: 370 calories, 13 g fat, 2 g saturated fat, 42 g protein, 18 g carbohydrate, 3 g dietary fiber, 190 mg sodium

Chicken and Avocado Salad

PREP TIME: 20 minutes

Tangy lime, aromatic cilantro, and creamy avocado give this refreshing salad a deep Mexican flavor; chicken turns it into a satisfying one-dish meal for lunch or dinner.

3 tablespoons extra-virgin olive oil

2 tablespoons fresh lime juice

1 tablespoon chopped fresh cilantro

¼ teaspoon salt

1 (1-pound) head romaine lettuce, chopped (8 cups)

2 medium tomatoes, diced

1 medium cucumber, peeled, seeded, and sliced

1 pound cooked chicken breasts, shredded

1 avocado, pitted, peeled, and sliced

Freshly ground black pepper

Whisk together oil, lime juice, cilantro, salt, and a pinch or two of pepper in a small mixing bowl.

Combine lettuce, tomatoes, and cucumber in a large mixing bowl. Toss with half of the dressing and season to taste with salt and pepper; divide among 4 plates.

Toss chicken with 1 tablespoon of the remaining dressing and divide among salads. Top with avocado slices, drizzle with remaining dressing, and serve.

Makes 4 (3-cup) servings

NUTRITION AT A GLANCE

Per serving: 380 calories, 21 g fat, 3.5 g saturated fat, 38 g protein, 10 g carbohydrate, 5 g dietary fiber, 240 mg sodium

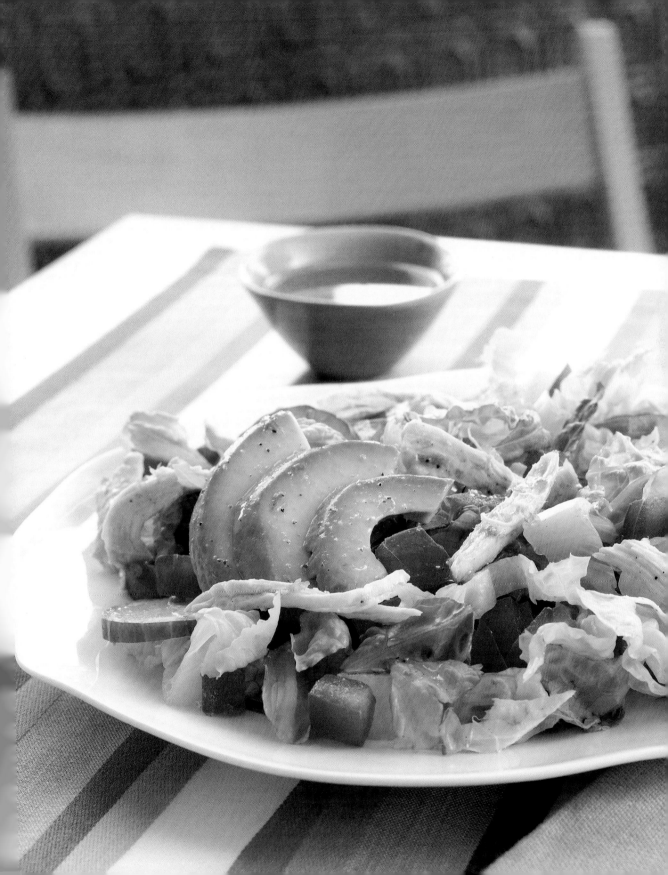

Chicken Pot Pie

PREP TIME: 10 minutes   **COOK TIME:** 30 minutes

Who would have thought that you could enjoy this classic favorite on the South Beach Diet? With our version, you can. The filling for this recipe can be made up to 3 days in advance and stored in the refrigerator. Warm it slightly before topping with the crust.

  2 tablespoons plus 2 teaspoons extra-virgin olive oil, divided

12 small white mushrooms, quartered

  1 small onion, diced

½ teaspoon dried thyme

1½ pounds boneless, skinless chicken breasts, cut into ½-inch cubes

  1 cup lower-sodium chicken broth

  1 tablespoon cornstarch

½ cup fat-free half-and-half

½ cup frozen peas and carrots

  4 sheets whole-wheat phyllo dough

    Salt and freshly ground black pepper

Heat oven to 400°F.

Heat 2 teaspoons of the oil in a large straight-sided skillet over medium heat. Add mushrooms and onion; cook until lightly browned and softened, about

5 minutes. Add thyme and chicken; cook until chicken is firm and cooked through, about 5 minutes.

Whisk together broth and cornstarch; add broth mixture and half-and-half to skillet. Bring mixture to a simmer and cook until slightly thickened, about 2 minutes. Stir in peas and carrots, reduce heat to low, and cook 2 minutes. Season with salt and pepper to taste and pour mixture into a 9-inch ovenproof pie dish.

Pour remaining 2 tablespoons oil into a small bowl. Lay 1 phyllo sheet on a clean work surface. Quickly brush the surface with a small amount of oil. Top with a second sheet and brush with more oil. Repeat with remaining sheets and oil.

Place phyllo over filling. Using scissors, trim excess phyllo, leaving a 1-inch border of overhanging dough. Fold dough in toward the center and pinch together to create an edge. Cut a small slit in the center of the phyllo to allow steam to escape during baking. Bake until golden and crisp, about 15 minutes.

Makes 6 servings

NUTRITION AT A GLANCE

Per serving: 260 calories, 9 g fat, 1.5 g saturated fat, 30 g protein, 14 g carbohydrate, 1 g dietary fiber, 230 mg sodium

Chicken Green Curry

PREP TIME: 15 minutes   **COOK TIME:** 20 minutes

If you thought making a quick Thai curry at home was impossible, think again! With some store-bought curry paste, made from green chilies, lemongrass, and kaffir lime, you'll be putting together an authentic, home-cooked curry in a jiffy. Look for the paste in the Asian foods section of your market. Serve this dish with sautéed vegetables or, in Phase 2 or 3, with brown rice.

1 (½-pound) bunch spinach (6 cups)

2 teaspoons canola oil

1 small onion, roughly chopped

1 (13.5-ounce) can light coconut milk

¼ cup lower-sodium chicken broth

1 tablespoon green curry paste (from a jar)

¼ teaspoon salt

1½ pounds boneless, skinless chicken breasts, sliced into thin strips

1 (1-pound) eggplant, cut into 1-inch cubes

2 tablespoons fresh lime juice

Cut tough stems from spinach; submerge in cold water and rinse thoroughly to remove any dirt.

Heat oil in a large straight-sided skillet over medium-high heat. Add onion and cook, stirring often, until softened, about 5 minutes. Stir in coconut milk, broth, curry paste, and salt; bring to a boil, reduce heat, and simmer for 8 minutes.

Add chicken and eggplant; bring to a low boil, then reduce to a simmer and cook, stirring occasionally, until chicken is no longer pink inside and eggplant is tender, about 8 minutes. Add spinach, stir, and cook 1 minute more. Stir in lime juice and serve.

Makes 4 (1¼-cup) servings

NUTRITION AT A GLANCE

Per serving: 340 calories, 12 g fat, 6 g saturated fat, 44 g protein, 15 g carbohydrate, 5 g dietary fiber, 400 mg sodium

Turkey Noodle Soup

PREP TIME: 10 minutes   **COOK TIME:** 20 minutes

Make this soup when you're craving a soul-satisfying bowl of comfort. Spelt noodles have a delicious nutty flavor and are high in fiber, protein, and B vitamins. You can also use whole-wheat noodles.

2 teaspoons extra-virgin olive oil

1 small onion, roughly chopped

1 carrot, diced

1 celery stalk, diced

1 garlic clove, minced

1 pound turkey cutlets, diced

5 cups lower-sodium chicken broth

1 teaspoon dried thyme

4 ounces spelt or whole-wheat noodles

Salt and freshly ground black pepper

Heat oil in a large saucepan over medium-high heat. Add onion, carrot, and celery; cook, stirring often, until softened, 5 minutes. Add garlic and cook 1 minute more.

Season turkey with salt and pepper. Add turkey, broth, and thyme to the onion mixture and bring to a low boil. Reduce heat to medium-low, cover, and simmer 5 minutes.

Stir in noodles, bring to a low boil, and cook until

noodles are tender, about 5 minutes more. Season to taste with salt and pepper and serve hot.

Makes 4 (2-cup) servings

NUTRITION AT A GLANCE

Per serving: 300 calories, 5 g fat, 1 g saturated fat, 38 g protein, 27 g carbohydrate, 4 g dietary fiber, 280 mg sodium

Baked Barbecue Chicken

PREP TIME: 10 minutes   **COOK TIME:** 25 minutes

Enjoy tangy barbecue any time of the year with this simple oven-baked dish. Serve it with Eggless Caesar Salad (page 161) or in Phase 2 or 3 with Moroccan Cabbage and Carrot Slaw (page 177).

4 (6-ounce) boneless, skinless chicken breasts

1 teaspoon extra-virgin olive oil

½ cup South Beach Barbecue Sauce (opposite page)

Salt and freshly ground black pepper

Heat oven to 350°F.

Season chicken on both sides with salt and pepper. Heat oil in a large nonstick skillet over medium-high heat. Add chicken and cook until browned, 2 minutes per side.

Place chicken, in a single layer, in an ovenproof baking dish and spoon sauce evenly over the top. Bake until chicken is cooked through and sauce is bubbling, 18 to 20 minutes.

Makes 4 servings

NUTRITION AT A GLANCE

Per serving: 200 calories, 3.5 g fat, .5 g saturated fat, 40 g protein, 2 g carbohydrate, 0 g dietary fiber, 290 mg sodium

South Beach Barbecue Sauce

PREP TIME: 10 minutes

This zesty sauce can be quickly made from scratch with a few basic pantry items. Store it in the refrigerator for up to 1 week.

1 (8-ounce) can tomato sauce

2 tablespoons white vinegar

2 teaspoons chopped fresh parsley

1 teaspoon Worcestershire sauce

1 teaspoon ground mustard

¼ teaspoon salt

⅛ teaspoon freshly ground black pepper

⅛ teaspoon garlic powder

Combine tomato sauce, vinegar, parsley, Worcestershire sauce, mustard, salt, pepper, and garlic powder in a resealable plastic container. Refrigerate until ready to use.

Makes 4 (¼-cup) servings

NUTRITION AT A GLANCE

Per serving: 25 calories, 0 g fat, 0 g saturated fat, 1 g protein, 5 g carbohydrate, 1 g dietary fiber, 380 mg sodium

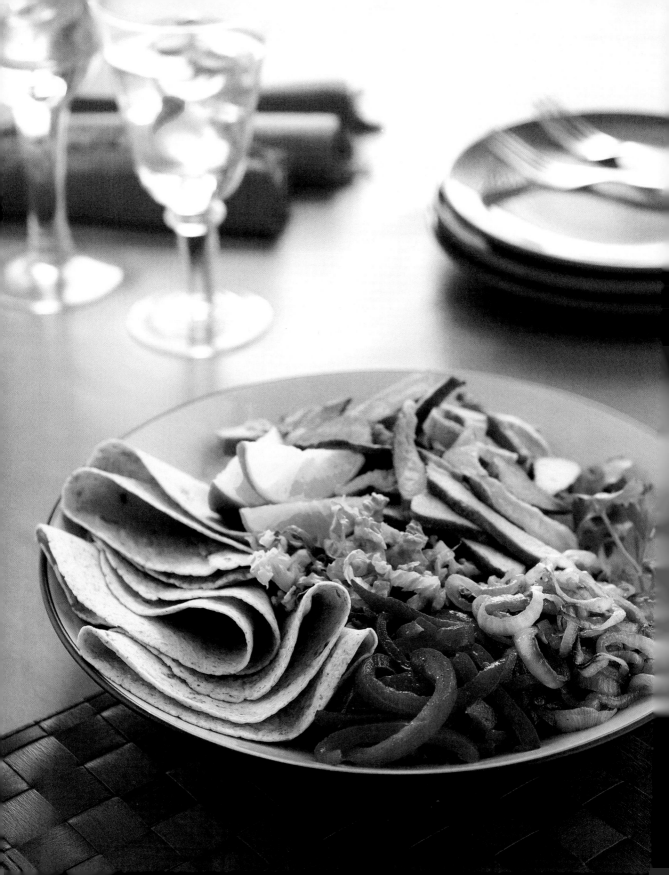

BEEF, PORK, AND LAMB

There's no reason that meat can't be part of a heart-healthy diet, but choosing the right cuts is a big part of the equation. Stick to the suggestions in this chapter, including tasty sirloin and top or bottom round steak, and you won't go wrong. If you have the opportunity, try grass-fed beef. It tastes great and is generally lower in saturated fat.

You'll find meatballs, kebabs, steaks, chops, and cutlets, such as Grilled Ancho-Rubbed Flank Steaks, Veal Piccata, Stuffed Pork Burgers, and Yogurt-Marinated Lamb Kebabs, in the pages ahead. Preparing plain meats thoughtfully using healthy extra-virgin olive oil will allow you to enjoy them with delicious, quick-to-prepare accompaniments, like tasty Asian dip, tangy mustard sauce, and tender peppers and onions.

◄ *Pork Fajitas (page 312)*

Pork Fajitas

PREP TIME: 10 minutes   COOK TIME: 25 minutes

Eat these tasty fajitas as is or top them with chopped lettuce, fresh cilantro, or salsa.

     4 (8-inch) whole-wheat tortillas

     1 tablespoon plus 2 teaspoons fresh lime juice, divided

     1 tablespoon plus 1½ teaspoons extra-virgin olive oil, divided

     1 garlic clove, minced

     1 teaspoon chili powder

  1½ pounds pork cutlets, about ½ inch thick

     1 large red bell pepper, cut into thin strips

     1 small onion, thinly sliced

       Salt and freshly ground black pepper

Heat oven or toaster oven to 200°F. Roll tortillas in foil and place in oven to warm.

Whisk together 1 tablespoon of the lime juice, 1 tablespoon of the oil, garlic, and chili powder in a large mixing bowl. Add pork and stir to coat. Cover with plastic wrap and marinate at room temperature for 15 minutes.

While pork is marinating, heat remaining oil in a medium nonstick skillet over medium-high heat. Add bell pepper and onion. Cook, stirring occasionally, until vegetables are softened and lightly browned, 10 to 12 minutes. Add remaining lime juice, stir, and remove from heat; season with salt and pepper. Transfer to a plate and cover loosely with foil to keep warm. Wipe pan dry with paper towels.

Season pork on both sides with salt and pepper. Heat the same skillet over high heat. Cook pork until no longer pink in the center, about 4 minutes per side. Transfer to a cutting board and let rest for 2 minutes.

Slice pork into thin strips, place on a platter with peppers and onions, and serve with warmed tortillas.

Makes 4 servings

NUTRITION AT A GLANCE

Per serving: 450 calories, 18 g fat, 4 g saturated fat, 41 g protein, 27 g carbohydrate, 3 g dietary fiber, 340 mg sodium

Rosemary Pork Medallions with Chunky Applesauce

PREP TIME: 5 minutes   **COOK TIME: 25 minutes**

Once you discover how easy it is to make a heavenly savory applesauce, the sauce alone might become a household staple. Pair it with our rosemary pork medallions and you've got a dinner the kids will love. The applesauce is great with roast chicken, too.

- 3 teaspoons extra-virgin olive oil, divided
- 1 small onion, diced
- 3 McIntosh apples (or other sweet variety), peeled, cored, and diced
- 1 tablespoon balsamic vinegar
- 3 tablespoons water
- 1½ pounds pork tenderloin, cut into medallions, about ¾ inch thick
- 2 teaspoons dried rosemary

  Salt and freshly ground black pepper

Heat 2 teaspoons of the oil in a medium skillet over medium heat. Add onion and cook until softened, about 3 minutes. Add apples, vinegar, and water; reduce heat to low and cook until tender, about 10 minutes. Remove from heat.

Season pork with rosemary, salt, and pepper. Heat remaining oil in a large nonstick skillet. Add pork and cook 4 minutes per side; remove from pan and serve with applesauce.

Makes 4 servings

NUTRITION AT A GLANCE

Per serving: 360 calories, 13 g fat, 4 g saturated fat, 36 g protein, 24 g carbohydrate, 4 g dietary fiber, 160 mg sodium

South Beach Classic Burger

PREP TIME: 10 minutes   **COOK TIME:** 10 minutes

Burger lovers, look out! Here is our version of the great American favorite. Look for ripe tomatoes at the peak of the season for an extra-juicy touch. Serve on whole-grain buns in Phases 2 and 3.

- 1½ pounds lean ground beef
- ¼ teaspoon salt
- ½ teaspoon freshly ground black pepper
- 2 ounces low-fat Swiss cheese slices
- 4 teaspoons Dijon mustard
- 4 green leaf lettuce leaves
- 1 medium tomato, sliced
- 1 small red onion, thinly sliced

Heat grill or grill pan to medium-high.

Mix together beef, salt, and pepper; form into 4 patties. Grill patties to desired doneness, 4 minutes per side for medium. Top with cheese and cover; cook until cheese is melted, 1 minute.

Remove from heat, spread with mustard, and top with lettuce, tomato, and onion; serve.

Makes 4 servings

NUTRITION AT A GLANCE

Per serving: 330 calories, 16 g fat, 6 g saturated fat, 39 g protein, 5 g carbohydrate, 0 g dietary fiber, 470 mg sodium

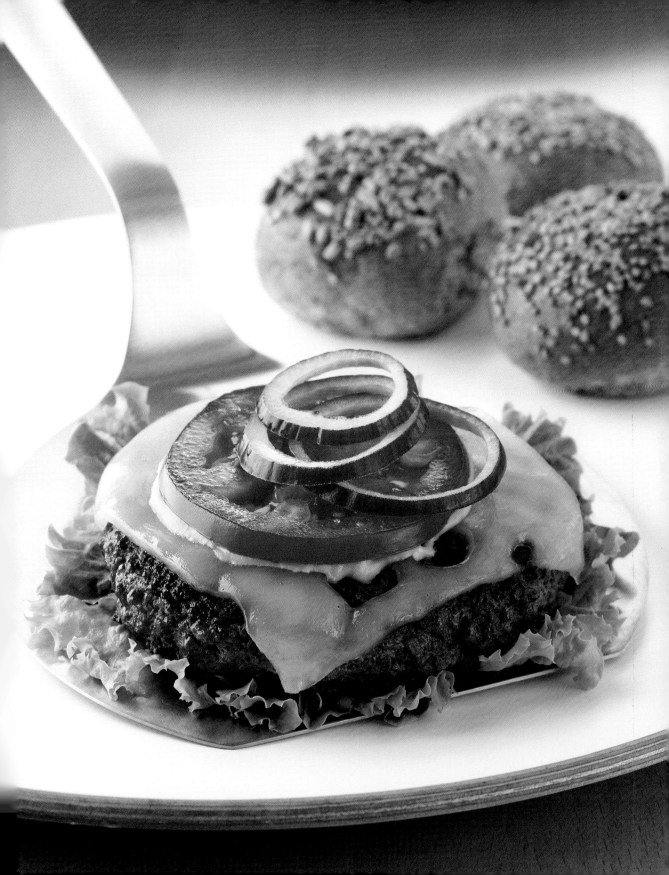

Thai Grilled Beef with String Beans

PREP TIME: 10 minutes   **COOK TIME:** 20 minutes

Made with fresh tangy lime and peppery chili paste, this restaurant favorite is surprisingly easy to make at home. Fish sauce (nuoc nam or nam pla) sounds very exotic but it is a common Southeast Asian condiment; look for it in the Asian section of your supermarket or health food store. Fresh mint can be used in place of cilantro—or try a mixture of both herbs. Top with chopped peanuts, if desired, for an authentic final touch.

1½ pounds flank steak

2 teaspoons extra-virgin olive oil, divided

¼ cup fresh lime juice

1 tablespoon Asian fish sauce (see page 27)

¼ teaspoon chili paste or 1 teaspoon seeded, minced serrano chile

1 teaspoon granular sugar substitute

1 cup coarsely chopped fresh cilantro

½ cup thinly sliced scallions

1 pound green beans, trimmed

Salt and freshly ground black pepper

Heat grill or grill pan to high. Rub steak on both sides with 1 teaspoon of the oil and season with salt and pepper. Grill until desired doneness, about 4 minutes per side for medium-rare. Remove from heat and set on a cutting board for 5 minutes.

Whisk together lime juice, fish sauce, chili paste, sugar substitute, cilantro, and scallions in a large mixing bowl.

Heat a saucepan of salted water until boiling. Add beans and cook until crisp-tender, about 3 minutes. Drain.

Thinly slice meat across the grain. Toss with lime juice mixture, adding any meat juices that have accumulated on the cutting board; add beans, toss, and serve.

Makes 4 servings

NUTRITION AT A GLANCE

Per serving: 340 calories, 17 g fat, 6 g saturated fat, 38 g protein, 10 g carbohydrate, 3 g dietary fiber, 530 mg sodium

Whole-Wheat Spaghetti with Ham and Peas

PREP TIME: 5 minutes   **COOK TIME: 25 minutes**

Salty ham and sweet peas are just part of the creamy sauce that makes this spaghetti sing. Be sure to scoop out some pasta cooking liquid before draining the pasta—this great trick gives the sauce extra body and flavor. Crushing dried basil with your fingers before adding it to the dish will release its full flavor.

- 8 ounces whole-wheat spaghetti
- 1½ teaspoons extra-virgin olive oil
- ½ small onion, finely chopped
- 1 teaspoon dried basil
- ⅛ teaspoon red pepper flakes
- 2 ounces thinly sliced lean ham, sliced into thin strips
- ¾ cup fat-free half-and-half
- 1 cup frozen peas, thawed
- 3 tablespoons freshly grated Parmesan cheese
- Salt and freshly ground black pepper

Cook pasta according to package directions. Before draining, reserve ½ cup of the pasta cooking liquid. Drain and set aside.

While pasta is cooking, heat oil in a large high-sided skillet over medium heat. Add onion, basil, and red pepper flakes. Cook until onions are translucent, about 2 minutes.

Add ham, half-and-half, and pasta cooking liquid. Bring to a simmer and cook until flavors blend and sauce thickens slightly, about 3 minutes.

Add peas and a good pinch of salt and pepper; cook for 2 minutes. Add pasta, toss to coat, reduce heat to low, and cook 1 minute more. Season with salt and pepper and serve hot with cheese.

Makes 4 (1½-cup) servings

NUTRITION AT A GLANCE

Per serving: 310 calories, 5 g fat, 1.5 g saturated fat, 16 g protein, 53 g carbohydrate, 9 g dietary fiber, 430 mg sodium

Mini Greek Meatballs

PREP TIME: 10 minutes   **COOK TIME:** 20 minutes

Serve these Mediterranean meatballs with roasted vegetables or a big Greek salad. In later phases, try them with Bulgur, Cucumber, and Mint Salad (page 167) topped with a generous handful of chopped fresh parsley or mint. To get ahead: Freeze just-shaped meatballs on a plate in a single layer for 1 hour, then transfer frozen meatballs to a labeled, resealable plastic bag. When you're ready to enjoy them, the meatballs will be too. Just cook them straight from the freezer, following the directions below.

- 1 pound lean ground beef
- ½ small onion, minced
- ½ cup finely crumbled reduced-fat feta cheese
- 2 garlic cloves, minced
- 1 large egg
- 1 tablespoon extra-virgin olive oil, plus more for baking dish
- 1 tablespoon dried oregano
- 1 tablespoon plus 1 teaspoon red wine vinegar
- ¼ teaspoon salt
- ¼ teaspoon freshly ground black pepper

Heat oven to 400°F.

Combine beef, onion, cheese, garlic, egg, 1 tablespoon oil, oregano, vinegar, salt, and pepper in a large mixing bowl. Knead to combine, being careful not to overmix.

Lightly oil a 9- by 13-inch baking dish. Shape meat mixture into 40 (1-tablespoon) meatballs. Place in a single layer in the baking dish and bake until cooked through, 12 to 15 minutes. Serve hot.

Makes 4 (10-piece) servings

NUTRITION AT A GLANCE

Per serving: 260 calories, 14 g fat, 5 g saturated fat, 30 g protein, 4 g carbohydrate, 0 g dietary fiber, 480 mg sodium

Yogurt-Marinated Lamb Kebabs

PREP TIME: 25 minutes (includes marinating)
COOK TIME: 15 minutes

This tangy, garlicky grilled lamb dish—with charred peppers and onion—brings the taste of Greece to your table in no time. To help save time, look for cut lamb at the butcher shop or supermarket and grill the veggies and lamb simultaneously so all the components of the dish are ready at once. Serve with Feta, Cucumber, and Radish Salad (page 172) or, in later phases, with Quinoa Pilaf (page 418).

1½ pounds well-trimmed boneless leg of lamb, cut into 2-inch cubes

½ cup plain fat-free or low-fat yogurt

2 garlic cloves, minced

2 medium green bell peppers, cut into 1-inch squares

1 medium onion, cut into wedges

1 tablespoon extra-virgin olive oil, plus extra for grill

Salt and freshly ground black pepper

Special equipment:

Skewers (if wooden, soak in water for 30 minutes)

Place lamb in a mixing bowl. Season generously with salt and pepper, add yogurt and garlic, and toss to combine. Cover bowl with plastic wrap and marinate at room temperature for 15 minutes.

While lamb is marinating, heat grill or grill pan to medium-high. Place bell peppers and onion in a mixing bowl, toss with oil, and season with salt and pepper. Thread vegetables onto skewers. Brush grill with oil and grill vegetables until browned, turning occasionally, about 15 minutes.

Place lamb on skewers and grill 4 minutes per side for medium-rare or 5 minutes per side for medium. Serve lamb with vegetables.

Makes 4 servings

NUTRITION AT A GLANCE

Per serving: 300 calories, 13 g fat, 4.5 g saturated fat, 37 g protein, 8 g carbohydrate, 1 g dietary fiber, 230 mg sodium

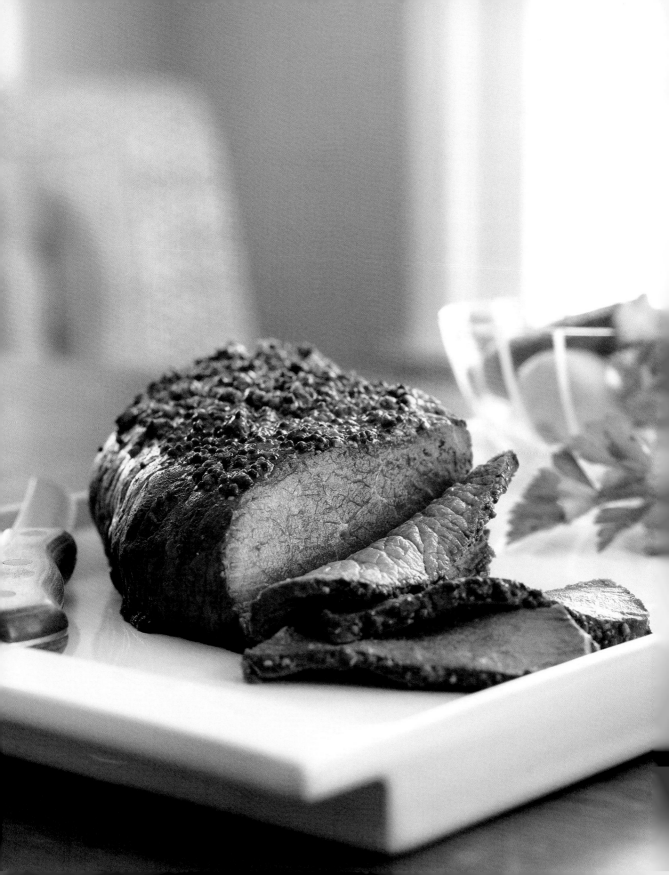

Mustard-Crusted Steak

PREP TIME: 15 minutes (includes marinating)
COOK TIME: 15 minutes

Two kinds of mustard and a generous measure of garlic give subtle flavor to this easy steak. Let the meat rest after cooking and slice it as thinly as possible for maximum tenderness. Pair this dish with Stuffed Baked Tomatoes (page 414) or Spinach with Garlic and Pine Nuts (page 437); in later phases, try it with Nutty Brown Rice (page 421).

2 garlic cloves, minced

1 tablespoon coarse-grain Dijon mustard

1 tablespoon Worcestershire sauce

1 teaspoon ground mustard

⅛ teaspoon salt

½ teaspoon freshly ground black pepper

1½ pounds boneless top round steak, ¾ inch thick

Heat oven to broil.

Whisk together garlic, Dijon mustard, Worcestershire sauce, ground mustard, salt, and pepper in a small mixing bowl.

Line a broiler pan with foil and place steak on top. Coat evenly with mustard mixture and let stand

10 minutes. Broil steak to desired doneness, 4 minutes per side for medium-rare. Let stand 5 minutes before slicing and serving.

Makes 4 servings

NUTRITION AT A GLANCE

Per serving: 250 calories, 9 g fat, 3 g saturated fat, 39 g protein, 2 g carbohydrate, 0 g dietary fiber, 260 mg sodium

Grilled Stuffed Veal Chops

PREP TIME: 15 minutes   **COOK TIME:** 10 minutes

Because veal chops can be an expensive treat, you won't want to cover up their delicate flavor with heavy sauces. Instead, try stuffing them with this flavorful yet light Italian-style filling. You can also use pork chops for this recipe.

- 4 (8- to 10-ounce) bone-in veal chops, about 1 inch thick
- 2 teaspoons extra-virgin olive oil, plus extra for grill
- ⅛ teaspoon salt
- ⅛ teaspoon freshly ground black pepper
- ¼ cup crumbled reduced-fat feta cheese (1 ounce)
- ¼ cup chopped roasted red bell peppers (from a jar)
- 1 teaspoon dried basil

Heat grill or grill pan to medium-high.

With a sharp paring knife, carefully cut a slit into the side of 1 veal chop to make a pocket for the filling, leaving a 1-inch border on three sides. Repeat with remaining chops. Rub chops with 2 teaspoons oil and season with salt and pepper.

Combine cheese, bell peppers, and basil in a small bowl. Spoon about 2 tablespoons into each chop. Brush grill with oil and grill chops 5 minutes per side for medium. Serve hot.

Makes 4 servings

NUTRITION AT A GLANCE

Per serving: 250 calories, 9 g fat, 3 g saturated fat, 39 g protein, 1 g carbohydrate, 0 g dietary fiber, 270 mg sodium

Sirloin Steak with Artichokes, Tomatoes, and Olives

PREP TIME: 10 minutes   **COOK TIME:** 20 minutes

Redolent with the lusty flavors of the Mediterranean, this dish turns a quick weeknight meal into something the whole family will look forward to coming home to. Serve it with your favorite salad. If you don't have time to thaw frozen artichokes, use a 14-ounce can of brine-packed ones, drained.

- 4 (6-ounce) sirloin steaks, about ¾ inch thick
- 2 teaspoons extra-virgin olive oil
- ¼ cup water
- 1 garlic clove, minced
- 1 teaspoon dried oregano
- 4 plum tomatoes, diced
- 1 (9-ounce) package frozen artichoke hearts, thawed and quartered
- ½ cup pitted kalamata olives, coarsely chopped

  Salt and freshly ground black pepper

Season steaks with salt and pepper. Heat oil in a large skillet over medium-high heat. Cook steak 4 to 5 minutes per side for medium-rare. Transfer to a plate.

Add water to the hot pan, scraping any brown bits from the bottom; reduce heat to medium. Add garlic and oregano; cook until garlic has softened, about

1 minute. Add tomatoes and cook 3 minutes more. Stir in artichokes and olives and cook until warmed through, about 2 minutes. Season with salt and pepper to taste and serve warm with steaks.

Makes 4 servings

NUTRITION AT A GLANCE

Per serving: 310 calories, 14 g fat, 3.5 g saturated fat, 40 g protein, 9 g carbohydrate, 5 g dietary fiber, 320 mg sodium

Vietnamese Pork Rolls

PREP TIME: 15 minutes   **COOK TIME:** 20 minutes
(includes assembling rolls)

These rolls are special, yet not hard to make. A simply dressed green salad with cucumber or radish would be a perfect accompaniment. Cut them on the diagonal or cut the lettuce leaves into thirds and roll up smaller, hors d'oeuvre-size pieces.

Dressing:

- 1 tablespoon Asian fish sauce (page 27)
- 1 tablespoon fresh lime juice
- 2 teaspoons minced fresh ginger
- 1 garlic clove, minced

    Pinch red pepper flakes

Pork:

- 1 tablespoon canola oil
- 1 pound pork cutlets
- 1 (½-pound) head napa cabbage, shredded (3 cups)
- 1 small red bell pepper, cut into thin strips
- 8 large Boston lettuce leaves

    Salt and freshly ground black pepper

For the dressing: Whisk together fish sauce, lime juice, ginger, garlic, and red pepper flakes in a small bowl.

For the pork: Heat oil in a large skillet over medium heat. Season pork with salt and pepper and sauté until lightly browned, 3 minutes per side. Remove from heat and slice into thin strips. Toss with 1 tablespoon of the dressing.

Combine cabbage, bell pepper, and remaining dressing in a large bowl. Lay lettuce leaves on a clean, dry work surface. Divide pork among leaves. Top with cabbage mixture and roll tightly, tucking edges in as you go. Place rolls, seam side down, on a cutting board, cut in half, and serve.

Makes 4 servings

NUTRITION AT A GLANCE

Per serving: 220 calories, 10 g fat, 2.5 g saturated fat, 26 g protein, 6 g carbohydrate, 2 g dietary fiber, 490 mg sodium

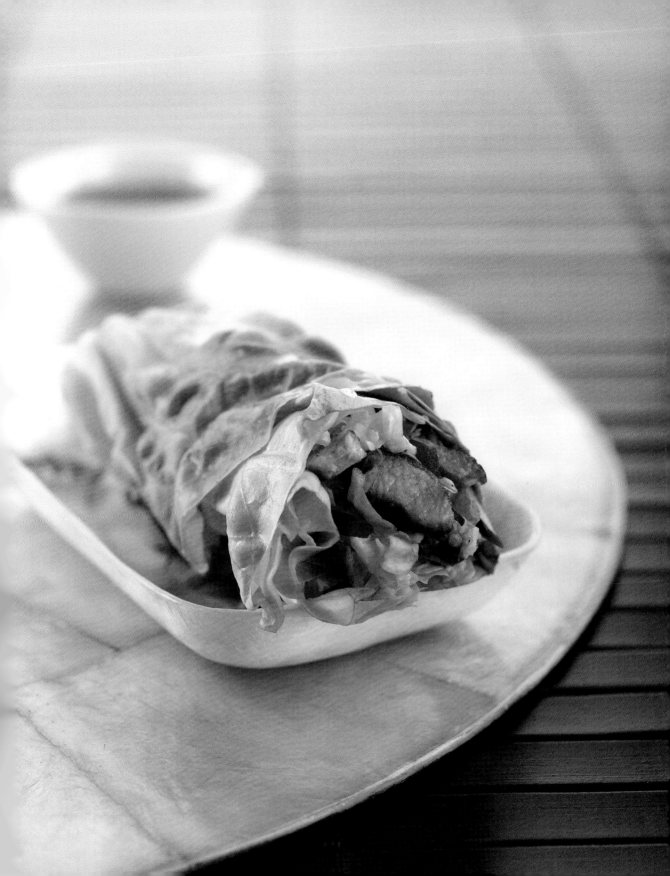

Grilled Ancho-Rubbed Flank Steak

PREP TIME: 20 minutes (includes marinating)
COOK TIME: 15 minutes

When fresh poblano chilies ripen and dry, they're called anchos. You'll find ground ones in a well-stocked supermarket, or you can buy them whole and grind them in a spice grinder. Serve this tangy, mildly spicy steak with your favorite salsa or, in later phases, use it to make fajitas with grilled vegetables and whole wheat tortillas.

> 1½ pounds flank steak, 1 inch thick
> 2 teaspoons ground ancho chili pepper
> ¼ teaspoon salt
> 2 teaspoons extra-virgin olive oil
> 2 teaspoons grated lime zest
> 1 tablespoon fresh lime juice
> Lime wedges

Heat grill or grill pan to high.

Season steak with chili pepper and salt. Combine oil, lime zest, and lime juice in a shallow dish and stir to mix well. Add steak and turn to coat. Let marinate at room temperature for 15 minutes.

Grill steak until desired doneness, about 4 minutes per side for medium-rare. Let stand 5 minutes before cutting into thin slices. Serve with lime wedges.

Makes 4 servings

NUTRITION AT A GLANCE

Per serving: 310 calories, 17 g fat, 6 g saturated fat, 36 g protein, 1 g carbohydrate, 0 g dietary fiber, 240 mg sodium

T-Bone Steak with Gremolata

PREP TIME: 10 minutes   **COOK TIME:** 20 minutes

Gremolata, a traditional Italian garnish served with braised veal shanks and other meats, is a simple mix of garlic, lemon zest, and fresh parsley. It gives an ordinary steak a burst of vibrant flavor. Use two skillets, or the grill, to cook the steaks simultaneously, if you want all four to be ready at once—it also cuts your cooking time in half.

3 tablespoons chopped fresh parsley

2 garlic cloves, minced

2 teaspoons grated lemon zest

4 (1-pound) T-bone steaks, ¾ inch thick

Salt and freshly ground black pepper

Combine parsley, garlic, lemon zest, and a pinch of salt and pepper in a small mixing bowl. Refrigerate until ready to use (gremolata can be made up to 4 hours ahead).

Season steaks generously with salt and pepper. Heat a large skillet over medium-high heat. Add 2 steaks and cook 4 minutes per side for medium-rare; transfer to a plate, cover loosely with foil to keep warm, and repeat with remaining steaks. Serve with gremolata.

Makes 4 servings

NUTRITION AT A GLANCE

Per serving: 350 calories, 12 g fat, 4.5 g saturated fat, 56 g protein, 1 g carbohydrate, 0 g dietary fiber, 220 mg sodium

Pork Cutlets with Orange, Red Onion, and Rosemary

PREP TIME: 10 minutes   **COOK TIME:** 12 minutes

Orange and rosemary make a dynamic savory pair, bringing irresistible flavor to an easy-to-cook cut of pork. Cutlets are thin and lean, so they cook up in minutes. To ensure tenderness, be careful not to overcook.

8 (3-ounce) pork cutlets, about ¾ inch thick

¾ teaspoon dried rosemary

2 tablespoons extra-virgin olive oil, divided

1 tablespoon minced red onion

½ cup lower-sodium chicken broth

Grated zest and juice from 1 small orange

Salt and freshly ground black pepper

Season cutlets with salt and pepper and rub with rosemary. Heat 1 tablespoon of the oil in a large skillet over medium-high heat. Cook cutlets, in batches if necessary, until lightly browned, about 2 minutes per side. Transfer to a plate.

Reduce heat to low. Add remaining oil to the skillet. Add onion and cook 1 minute. Raise heat to medium-high; add broth and orange zest and juice and cook until liquid is reduced by half and slightly thickened, about 3 minutes. Add pork back to the skillet and cook, turning to coat; cook 1 minute more.

Makes 4 servings

NUTRITION AT A GLANCE

Per serving: 320 calories, 17 g fat, 4.5 g saturated fat, 37 g protein, 3 g carbohydrate, 0 g dietary fiber, 170 mg sodium

Beef and Bean Chili

PREP TIME: 5 minutes **COOK TIME: 25 minutes**

Top this hearty chili with chopped scallions, reduced-fat sour cream, or grated low-fat cheddar cheese.

- 1 tablespoon extra-virgin olive oil
- 1 pound lean ground beef
- 2½ teaspoons chili powder, divided
- 1 teaspoon ground cumin
- 1 small onion, thinly sliced
- 2 garlic cloves
- 1 (28-ounce) can diced tomatoes
- 1 (15-ounce) can kidney beans, rinsed and drained

  Salt and freshly ground black pepper

Heat oil in a large heavy-bottomed saucepan over medium-high heat. Add beef, 1 teaspoon of the chili powder, and cumin; sauté until browned, about 5 minutes. Using a slotted spoon, transfer beef to a plate.

Add onion, garlic, and remaining chili powder to the same saucepan; cook over medium heat, stirring occasionally, until softened, about 3 minutes. Add tomatoes with juice and beans; cover and simmer 10 minutes, stirring occasionally.

Uncover, add cooked beef, and cook an additional

5 minutes, until liquid thickens slightly. Season to taste with salt and pepper and serve hot.

Makes 4 (1½-cup) servings

NUTRITION AT A GLANCE

Per serving: 350 calories, 15 g fat, 4.5 g saturated fat, 30 g protein, 25 g carbohydrate, 8 g dietary fiber, 670 mg sodium

Warm Beef Salad

PREP TIME: 10 minutes   **COOK TIME:** 15 minutes

Smoky grilled beef, crisp greens, and a zippy lemon dressing make up this satisfying main-dish salad. Purchasing washed, packaged salad greens will help keep prep time quick.

- 1½ pounds flank steak, 1 inch thick
- 2 tablespoons fresh lemon juice
- 2 teaspoons grated lemon zest
- ½ teaspoon Dijon mustard
- 2 tablespoons extra-virgin olive oil
- 5 ounces mesclun greens (6 cups)
- 4 plum tomatoes, cut into wedges
- 2 ounces reduced-fat feta cheese, crumbled (½ cup)
- 1 small red onion, thinly sliced and separated into rings

Heat grill to high.

Grill steak 4 minutes per side for medium-rare. Let rest 5 minutes; slice thinly.

Place lemon juice, lemon zest, mustard, and oil in a jar with a lid. Close tightly and shake vigorously to combine. Place greens in a large mixing bowl, add 2 tablespoons of the dressing, and toss to coat.

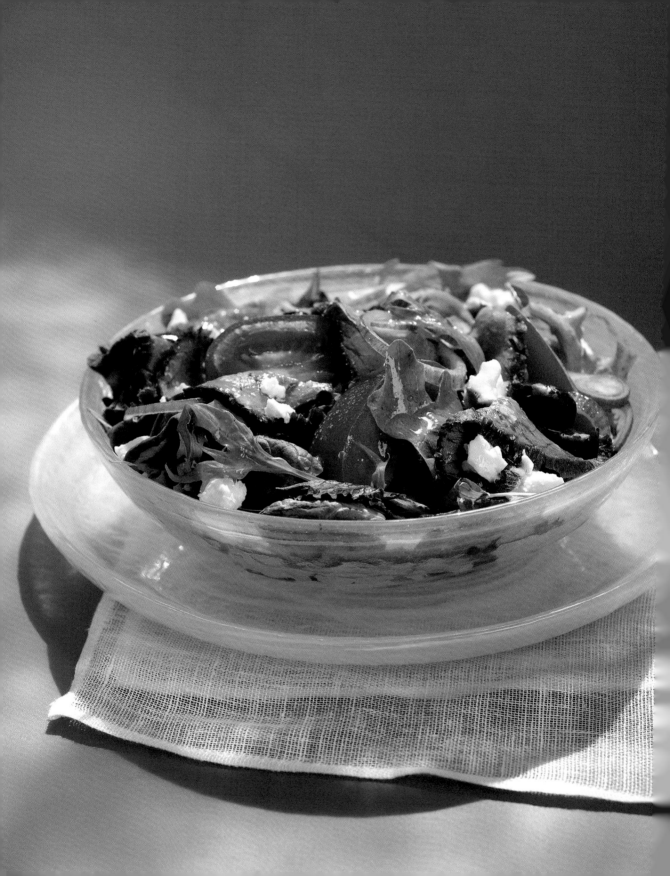

Divide greens among 4 serving plates, top with steak, tomato wedges, onion, and feta, and serve.

Makes 4 (2-cup) servings

NUTRITION AT A GLANCE

Per serving: 420 calories, 25 g fat, 9 g saturated fat, 42 g protein, 7 g carbohydrate, 2 g dietary fiber, 380 mg sodium

Santa Fe Steak

PREP TIME: 10 minutes   **COOK TIME:** 30 minutes

This fun twist on the usual steak and onions employs the heady flavors of the Southwest: cumin, garlic, and poblano peppers. If poblanos are not available, use a bell pepper (any color) and add a drop or two of hot sauce. If you have extra time, let the steak marinate at room temperature for 30 minutes for added flavor.

2 tablespoons extra-virgin olive oil, divided

1 large poblano pepper, sliced into ¼-inch strips

1 medium onion, thinly sliced

1 cup water

4 garlic cloves, minced

1 teaspoon ground cumin

1½ pounds flank steak

Salt and freshly ground black pepper

Heat 1 tablespoon of the oil in a nonstick skillet over medium-high heat. Add pepper strips and onion and cook, stirring occasionally, until softened and browned, about 8 minutes.

Add water, increase heat to high, and boil until liquid is almost evaporated and vegetables are tender, 4 minutes more. Remove from heat, season with salt and pepper, and cover to keep warm.

Heat grill or grill pan over medium-high heat. Mix garlic, cumin, and remaining oil together to form a thin paste. Spread over steak and rub well into both sides of the meat.

Season steak with salt and pepper and grill 5 minutes per side for medium-rare. Remove from heat, allow steak to rest for 5 minutes, and then thinly slice across the grain. Serve with peppers and onions.

Makes 4 servings

NUTRITION AT A GLANCE

Per serving: 310 calories, 15 g fat, 6 g saturated fat, 37 g protein, 6 g carbohydrate, 2 g dietary fiber, 170 mg sodium

Pork and Vegetable Stir-Fry

PREP TIME: 20 minutes   **COOK TIME: 10 minutes**

Apricot preserves give this stir-fry a subtly sweet, fruit finish reminiscent of those tasty Chinese sweet glazed dishes but without excessive sugars. Look for cut packaged veggies or "stir-fry mix" to lighten your workload and try chicken cutlets in place of pork, if you wish.

½ cup sugar-free apricot preserves

3 tablespoons low-sodium soy sauce

2 tablespoons canola oil, divided

1½ pounds pork cutlets, cut into ¼-inch strips

4 garlic cloves, minced

1 pound broccoli, cut into florets (3 to 4 cups)

1 red bell pepper, cut into thin strips

1 bunch scallions, cut into 2-inch lengths

4 ounces snow peas, strings removed

Whisk preserves and soy sauce together in a bowl until smooth.

Heat 1 tablespoon of the oil in a large nonstick skillet or wok over high heat. Add pork and cook, stirring frequently, until lightly browned and no longer pink, about 5 minutes. Transfer to a plate.

Add remaining oil and garlic to the same skillet; cook over medium-high heat for 30 seconds. Add broccoli, pepper, scallions, and snow peas and cook until vegetables are crisp-tender, about 3 minutes. Stir in pork and preserves mixture; cook 1 minute more. Serve hot.

Makes 4 (2-cup) servings

NUTRITION AT A GLANCE

Per serving: 400 calories, 17 g fat, 4 g saturated fat, 43 g protein, 24 g carbohydrate, 6 g dietary fiber, 890 mg sodium

Lamb Chops with Chimichurri Sauce

PREP TIME: 10 minutes   **COOK TIME:** 10 minutes

Citrusy, garlicky chimichurri, a common Argentinean condiment for beef, is a delectable companion to juicy lamb chops. We use fresh parsley and dried oregano in ours, but you can also try adding fresh cilantro and mint, if you'd like.

8 (3-ounce) lamb chops, about ¾ inch thick

¼ cup extra-virgin olive oil, divided

⅓ cup fresh parsley leaves

2 garlic cloves, peeled

1 tablespoons fresh lemon juice

½ teaspoon dried oregano

¼ teaspoon red pepper flakes

Salt and freshly ground black pepper

Heat grill or grill pan to high. Rub lamb chops with 1 tablespoon of the oil and season with salt and pepper. Grill 3 minutes per side for medium-rare. Remove from heat, cover loosely with foil, and allow meat to rest.

While lamb is resting, combine remaining oil, parsley, garlic, lemon juice, oregano, and red pepper

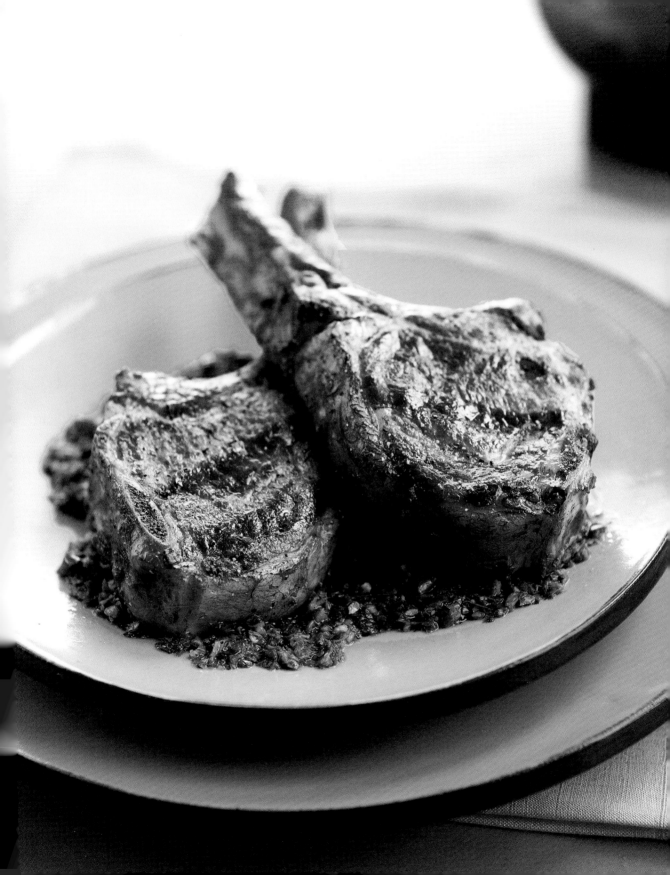

flakes in a food processor. Pulse to combine until just puréed. Season with salt and pepper and serve with lamb.

Makes 4 servings

NUTRITION AT A GLANCE

Per serving: 360 calories, 22 g fat, 5 g saturated fat, 35 g protein, 1 g carbohydrate, 0 g dietary fiber, 180 mg sodium

Veal Piccata

PREP TIME: 10 minutes   **COOK TIME:** 15 minutes

Tender golden veal perks up with a garlicky lemon and caper sauce in our version of a favorite classic.

1½ pounds veal cutlets, about ¼ inch thick

¼ cup whole-wheat flour

3 tablespoons extra-virgin olive oil, divided

2 garlic cloves, minced

½ cup lower-sodium chicken broth

⅓ cup fresh lemon juice

1½ tablespoons capers, rinsed and drained

2 tablespoons chopped fresh parsley

Salt and freshly ground black pepper

Season veal with salt and pepper. Place flour in a shallow dish and dredge veal to coat both sides; knock off excess flour.

Heat 1 tablespoon of the oil in a large nonstick skillet over medium-high heat. Add half of the veal and cook until lightly browned, 1½ minutes per side. Transfer to a platter and cover to keep warm. Repeat with remaining veal.

Heat remaining oil in the same skillet; add garlic and cook, stirring constantly, until fragrant, 30 seconds. Add broth and lemon juice; stir to scrape up the browned bits and bring to a boil. Cook until liquid is slightly reduced, about 2 minutes. Stir in capers and parsley. Add a pinch or two of pepper, drizzle sauce over veal, and serve.

Makes 4 servings

NUTRITION AT A GLANCE

Per serving: 300 calories, 14 g fat, 2.5 g saturated fat, 38 g protein, 6 g carbohydrate, 0 g dietary fiber, 220 mg sodium

Peppery Steak with Horseradish Cream

PREP TIME: 5 minutes   **COOK TIME: 20 minutes**

Steak lovers will enjoy this classic combination of smoky grilled meat and pungent horseradish. Leftovers make a great companion to salad or use them as sandwich fillings in later phases.

- 1½ pounds London broil or other sirloin steak (about 1 inch thick)
- 1 teaspoon extra-virgin olive oil
- 2 tablespoons cracked black pepper
- ½ cup reduced-fat sour cream
- 2 teaspoons prepared horseradish
- Salt

Rub steak with oil and pepper, pressing pepper into steak; season well with salt. Heat grill pan over medium-high heat or heat oven to broil. Grill or broil steak 5 to 6 minutes per side for medium-rare. Transfer to a cutting board and cover loosely with foil to keep warm. Allow meat to rest for 5 minutes before thinly slicing across the grain.

While steak is resting, mix together sour cream and horseradish; season to taste with salt. Serve horseradish cream with steak.

Makes 4 servings

NUTRITION AT A GLANCE

Per serving: 360 calories, 18 g fat, 8 g saturated fat, 39 g protein, 4 g carbohydrate, 0 g dietary fiber, 200 mg sodium

Beef with Asparagus and Mushrooms

PREP TIME: 10 minutes   **COOK TIME: 20 minutes**

Wood-scented rosemary, nutty garlic, and zesty lemon give an otherwise ordinary steak and vegetable dish a touch of sophistication. And here's a trick: Making shallow cuts in the steak before seasoning it gives the seasonings full access to the meat, resulting in deep, full flavor.

- 1½ pounds London broil, 1 inch thick
- 4 garlic cloves, minced, divided
- 4 teaspoons crushed dried rosemary, divided
- 2 tablespoons extra-virgin olive oil, divided
- 1 small onion, sliced lengthwise
- 1 pound asparagus, cut into 2-inch pieces
- 1 pound white mushrooms, sliced
- 2 teaspoons grated lemon zest
- Salt and freshly ground black pepper

Score both sides of steak in a diamond pattern by carefully making ⅛-inch-deep diagonal cuts with a sharp knife at 1-inch intervals. Rub half of the garlic and 2 teaspoons of the rosemary into both sides of meat and season with salt and pepper.

Heat 1 tablespoon of the oil in a large nonstick skillet over medium-high heat. Add steak and cook, turning once, about 4 minutes per side for medium-rare. Transfer to a plate and loosely cover with foil to keep warm.

Heat remaining oil in the same skillet. Add onion and cook, stirring often, for 2 minutes. Add remaining garlic and cook, stirring constantly, until fragrant, about 30 seconds. Add asparagus and mushrooms and cook, stirring often, until asparagus is crisp-tender and almost all the liquid has evaporated, about 5 minutes. Stir in lemon zest and remaining rosemary; season to taste with salt and pepper.

Cut steak into thin slices and serve with the vegetables.

Makes 4 servings

NUTRITION AT A GLANCE

Per serving: 370 calories, 17 g fat, 4.5 g saturated fat, 42 g protein, 12 g carbohydrate, 3 g dietary fiber, 180 mg sodium

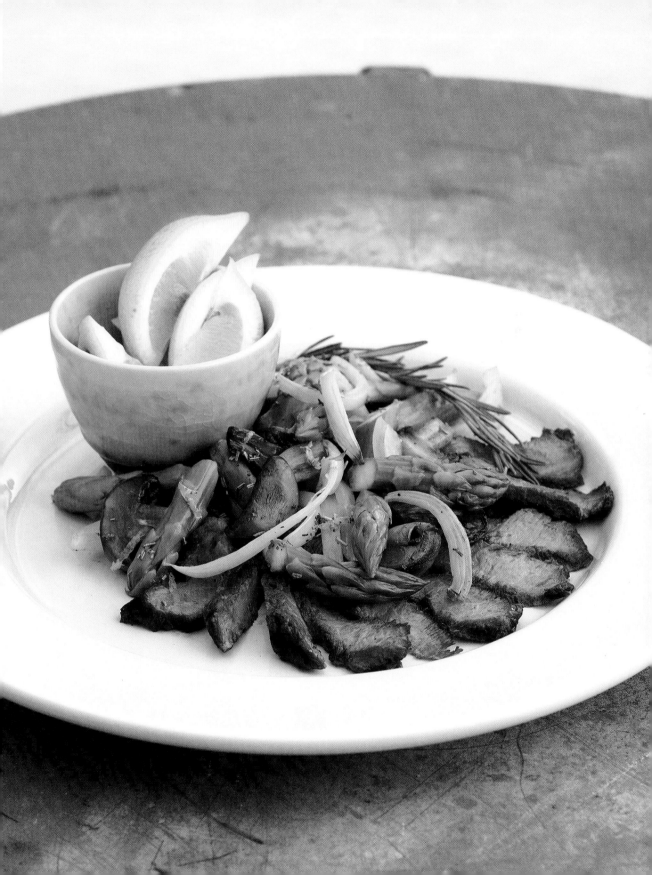

Pork Chops with Fennel and Lemon

PREP TIME: 5 minutes   **COOK TIME:** 20 minutes

Our quick lemony braise renders bone-in pork chops deliciously tender and tangy and makes delectable fennel subtly sweet.

4 (6-ounce) bone-in pork chops, about ½ inch thick

1 tablespoon extra-virgin olive oil

1 large fennel bulb, sliced into ½-inch strips

1 small onion, thinly sliced

1 cup lower-sodium chicken broth

2 tablespoons fresh lemon juice

Salt and freshly ground black pepper

Season pork chops with salt and pepper. Heat oil in a large skillet over medium-high heat. Cook pork chops until lightly browned, about 2 minutes per side. Transfer to a plate.

Add fennel and onion to the same skillet and cook until lightly browned and softened, about 3 minutes. Add broth and lemon juice, bring to a simmer, cover, and cook until fennel is crisp-tender, about 5 minutes. Uncover and simmer until liquid is reduced slightly, about 3 minutes.

Add pork back to the skillet and cook until heated through, about 2 minutes. Season with salt and pepper and serve hot.

Makes 4 servings

NUTRITION AT A GLANCE

Per serving: 300 calories, 19 g fat, 6 g saturated fat, 24 g protein, 7 g carbohydrate, 2 g dietary fiber, 170 mg sodium

Stuffed Pork Burger

PREP TIME: 10 minutes   **COOK TIME:** 10 minutes

These juicy, pesto-flavored burgers come with a delicious melted mozzarella surprise inside! Top them with lettuce and a slice of fresh, juicy tomato, if you'd like—or just enjoy them as is.

  5 tablespoons pesto (from a jar)

  ½ teaspoon salt

  1 teaspoon freshly ground black pepper

1½ pounds lean ground pork

  2 ounces low-fat mozzarella, cut into 4 cubes

Stir together pesto, salt, and pepper in a medium mixing bowl. Add pork and, using your hands, gently yet thoroughly combine; do not overmix.

Shape pork mixture into 4 equal-sized balls. Press 1 mozzarella cube into the center of each ball; gently form a ¾-inch-thick patty, enclosing the cheese.

Lightly coat a large nonstick skillet with cooking spray. Heat over medium-high heat. Add burgers, cooking in batches if necessary, reduce heat to medium, and cook 5 minutes per side. Serve hot.

Makes 4 servings

NUTRITION AT A GLANCE

Per serving: 380 calories, 22 g fat, 7 g saturated fat, 42 g protein, 1 g carbohydrate, 0 g dietary fiber, 620 mg sodium

Warm Steak Sandwich with Roasted Pepper Mayo

PREP TIME: 10 minutes   **COOK TIME: 5 minutes**

What could be more appropriate for a quick and easy cookbook than "minute steak," a very thin piece of boneless beefsteak named for its ability to cook up fast. Juicy and warm—and served in this succulent sandwich—it's one of our favorites.

  2 teaspoons extra-virgin olive oil

  1 pound top round steak, sliced into 8 pieces

  ¼ cup chopped roasted red pepper (from a jar)

  ¼ cup mayonnaise

  8 slices multigrain bread, lightly toasted

  1 small bunch arugula

    Salt and freshly ground black pepper

Heat oil in a large skillet over medium-high heat. Season steak with salt and pepper and cook until browned, about 2 minutes.

Purée red pepper and mayonnaise in a food processor until smooth. Spread mayonnaise on each slice of bread;

make sandwiches with steak slices and arugula. Slice each in half and serve.

Makes 4 servings

NUTRITION AT A GLANCE

Per serving: 380 calories, 20 g fat, 4 g saturated fat, 30 g protein, 21 g carbohydrate, 6 g dietary fiber, 490 mg sodium

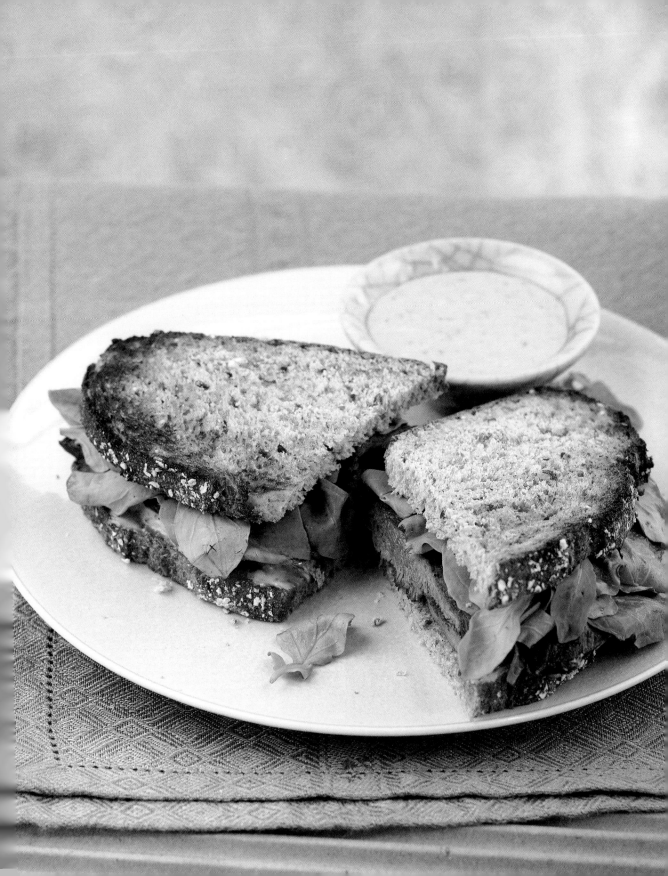

Beef and Bok Choy Fried Rice

PREP TIME: 10 minutes   **COOK TIME:** 15 minutes

We've "beefed up" traditional fried rice, trading some of the rice for added lean meat and vegetables and using brown rice instead of white.

2 tablespoons canola oil, divided

3 large eggs, lightly beaten

1½ pounds flank steak, cut into thin strips

1 tablespoon low-sodium soy sauce

2 scallions, sliced

2 garlic cloves, minced

1 tablespoon minced fresh ginger

1 (1½-pound) head bok choy, cut crosswise into ½-inch strips (6 to 7 cups)

2 cups cooked whole-grain quick-cooking brown rice (page 14)

Salt and freshly ground black pepper

Heat 1 tablespoon of the oil in a large skillet or wok over medium-high heat. Add eggs and swirl to cover bottom of pan, lifting edges with a heatproof spatula to let uncooked egg reach the bottom of the pan. Continue until egg is set, 1 minute. Remove egg from pan, slice, and set aside.

Season steak with salt and pepper, add to the same skillet, and cook over medium-high heat, stirring frequently, until browned, about 5 minutes. Transfer to a bowl, add soy sauce, and stir to combine.

Heat remaining oil in the skillet over medium-high heat. Add scallions, garlic, and ginger and cook for 1 minute. Add bok choy and cook, stirring occasionally, until crisp-tender, about 4 minutes. Add reserved beef, reserved egg, and rice; cook 2 minutes more. Serve hot.

Makes 4 (2-cup) servings

NUTRITION AT A GLANCE

Per serving: 490 calories, 21 g fat, 5 g saturated fat, 46 g protein, 27 g carbohydrate, 3 g dietary fiber, 540 mg sodium

Chipotle Beef Burrito

PREP TIME: 10 minutes   **COOK TIME:** 20 minutes

Canned chipotle peppers add smoke and a little heat to this quick-cooking beef and bean burrito.

- 2 teaspoons extra-virgin olive oil
- 1 small onion, diced
- 1 pound lean ground beef
- 2 canned chipotle chiles in adobo, chopped, plus 2 tablespoons sauce from can
- 1 (15-ounce) can black beans, rinsed and drained
- 1 (½-pound) bunch spinach, chopped (6 cups)
- 4 whole-wheat tortillas
- 2 ounces shredded reduced-fat cheddar cheese (½ cup)

  Salt and freshly ground black pepper

Heat oil in a large skillet over medium heat. Add onion and cook until softened, about 3 minutes. Add beef and cook until well browned, about 6 minutes; drain fat from pan.

Add chiles, adobo sauce, and beans to beef mixture; cook until beans are warmed through, about 3 minutes. Add spinach, cover, and cook until wilted, about 2 minutes. Season to taste with salt and pepper and remove from heat.

Heat tortillas in a skillet or microwave. Lay 1 tortilla on a serving plate. Top with ¼ cup of the cheese and 1 cup of the beef mixture. Fold two sides of the tortilla in toward the middle and roll up tortilla to form the burrito. Repeat with remaining filling and tortillas. Serve hot.

Makes 4 servings

NUTRITION AT A GLANCE

Per serving: 400 calories, 15 g fat, 4.5 g saturated fat, 34 g protein, 39 g carbohydrate, 8 g dietary fiber, 730 mg sodium

Pork Satay

PREP TIME: 5 minutes   **COOK TIME:** 15 minutes

Served with its own dipping sauce, this tasty satay dish turns dinner into a festive event. The pork can be broiled or grilled; if you don't have skewers, just broil the meat without them.

¼ cup creamy trans-fat-free peanut butter

¼ cup water

1 tablespoon plus 1½ teaspoons rice vinegar

2 tablespoons low-sodium soy sauce

2 garlic cloves, minced

⅛ teaspoon red pepper flakes

1½ pounds pork cutlets (about ¾ inch thick), cut lengthwise into ½-inch strips

Special equipment:

4 metal skewers

Heat oven to broil.

Whisk together peanut butter, water, vinegar, soy sauce, garlic, and red pepper flakes in a mixing bowl. Place pork in a separate mixing bowl, add 3 tablespoons of the peanut butter sauce, and toss to combine. Reserve remaining sauce.

Thread pork onto skewers and broil 4 minutes per side. Place remaining sauce in dipping cups and serve with pork.

Makes 4 servings

NUTRITION AT A GLANCE

Per serving: 360 calories, 18 g fat, 5 g saturated fat, 42 g protein, 5 g carbohydrate, 1 g dietary fiber, 420 mg sodium

Pork Scaloppine with Herbs

PREP TIME: 5 minutes   **COOK TIME:** 7 minutes

You'll love how just a couple of dried herbs, fresh lemon juice, and capers can transform simple pork cutlets into a vibrant, tangy dish that's great for a weeknight meal.

> 1½ pounds pork cutlets
>
> 1 teaspoon dried basil
>
> 1 teaspoon dried thyme
>
> 1 tablespoon extra-virgin olive oil
>
> 3 tablespoons fresh lemon juice
>
> 2 tablespoons capers, drained and rinsed
>
> Salt and freshly ground black pepper

Pound cutlets to ¼-inch thickness; rub with basil and thyme and season with salt and pepper.

Heat oil in a large nonstick skillet over medium-high heat. Add pork and cook 2 minutes per side. Remove to a plate and loosely cover with foil to keep warm.

Add lemon juice and capers to the skillet; bring to boil and cook until slightly reduced, about 1 minute. Top pork with sauce and serve hot.

Makes 4 servings

NUTRITION AT A GLANCE

Per serving: 290 calories, 14 g fat, 4 g saturated fat, 38 g protein, 1 g carbohydrate, 0 g dietary fiber, 280 mg sodium

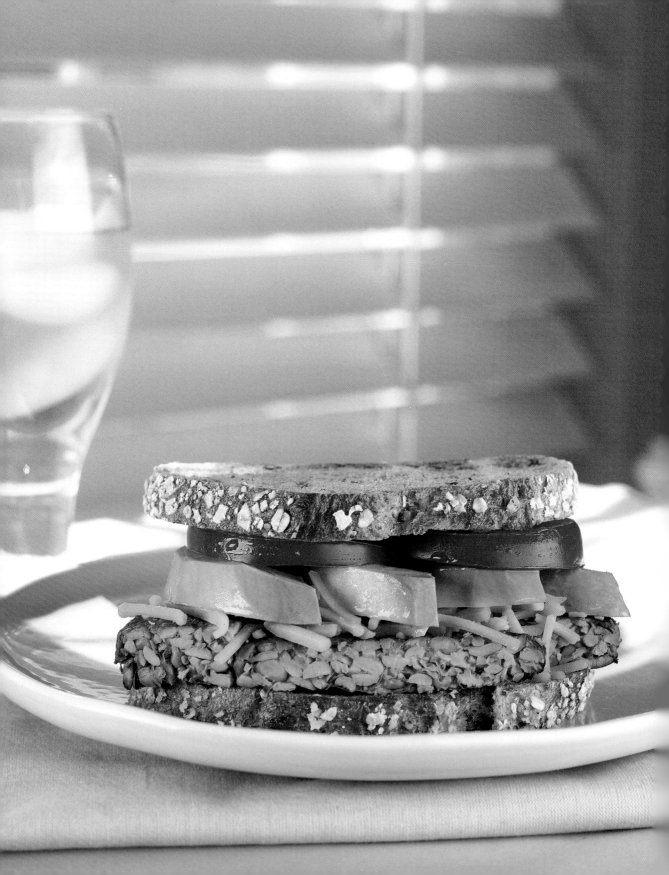

VEGETARIAN ENTRÉES

On the South Beach Diet, meals centered around vegetables and plant proteins go way beyond the usual stir-fries and veggie burgers.

We've put together an inspiring collection of dishes made with high protein staples that might even be new to longtime vegetarians. Ingredients like edamame (which are easily accessible year-round in the frozen foods section of most supermarkets), tempeh, and textured vegetable protein join tofu as central elements of delicious dishes that are free from processed carbs and not overly high in fat. Try Italian-Style Tofu Bake, Black Bean and Goat Cheese Tostadas, or Lentil and Kale Stew.

All of these dishes (including an irresistible macaroni and cheese) are high in flavor and low in prep time. Alongside protein-packed ingredients, you'll find fiber-rich foods like bulgur, kidney beans, and lentils.

◄ *Tempeh Dagwood Sandwich (page 374)*

Tempeh Dagwood Sandwich

PREP TIME: 15 minutes (includes marinating)
COOK TIME: 10 minutes

Stacked up high and filled with smooth avocado, juicy tomato, and creamy cheese, this power-protein sandwich is a South Beach vegetarian favorite. Vegans can use nondairy mayo and soy cheese. If you have extra time, marinate the tempeh for up to an hour.

- 2 tablespoons low-sodium soy sauce
- 1 tablespoon plus 1½ teaspoons cider vinegar
- 1 garlic clove, minced
- ½ (8-ounce) package soy tempeh
- 1 teaspoon mayonnaise
- 2 slices multigrain bread, lightly toasted
- 1 ounce shredded reduced-fat cheddar cheese (3 tablespoons)
- ¼ avocado, peeled and sliced
- 2 slices tomato

Whisk together soy sauce, vinegar, and garlic in a shallow bowl. Add tempeh and marinate for 10 minutes, turning once halfway through.

Spray a medium nonstick skillet with fat-free cooking spray and heat over medium heat. Add tempeh, reserving marinade, and cook until well browned,

4 minutes per side. Remove from heat, add 2 tablespoons of the marinade to the pan, and flip tempeh once or twice until marinade is absorbed.

Spread mayonnaise on 1 bread slice. Place tempeh on top and cover with cheese, avocado, and tomato. Top with remaining bread, gently press down, slice in half, and serve.

Makes 1 serving

NUTRITION AT A GLANCE

Per serving: 450 calories, 19 g fat, 5 g saturated fat, 37 g protein, 38 g carbohydrate, 16 g dietary fiber, 860 mg sodium

South Beach Macaroni and Cheese

PREP TIME: 5 minutes   **COOK TIME:** 30 minutes

Cheesy, creamy, rich, packed with protein, and low in fat, the South Beach version of "mac and cheese" is something to cheer about!

8 ounces spelt or whole-wheat elbow pasta

1 tablespoon trans-fat-free margarine

1 tablespoon whole-wheat flour

1¼ cups fat-free half-and-half

1 cup shredded reduced-fat sharp cheddar cheese

¼ teaspoon salt

⅛ teaspoon freshly ground black pepper

Heat oven to 400°F.

Bring a saucepan of salted water to a boil. Cook pasta until al dente (tender but still firm to the bite), about 6 minutes. Drain and rinse under cold water for 30 seconds.

While pasta is cooking, melt margarine in a wide, straight-sided skillet over medium heat. Add flour, reduce heat to low, and whisk continuously until flour is incorporated and cooked, about 2 minutes. Add half-and-half, bring to a simmer, and cook, whisking frequently, until blended and thickened, 3 to 5 minutes.

Add cheese, salt, and pepper; stir until blended. Add pasta and stir until coated and warmed, 1 minute. Transfer to an 8 by 8-inch baking dish and bake for 10 minutes. Serve hot.

Makes 4 (1½-cup) servings

NUTRITION AT A GLANCE

Per serving: 340 calories, 11 g fat, 5 g saturated fat, 17 g protein, 50 g carbohydrate, 5 g dietary fiber, 280 mg sodium

Tofu, Chickpea, and Sun-Dried Tomato Salad

PREP TIME: 10 minutes   **COOK TIME:** 15 minutes

This zesty Mediterranean salad combines protein from feta cheese, chickpeas, and tofu to make a filling meal.

- 1 (14-ounce) package extra-firm tofu, cut into ¼-inch slices
- ½ (1-pound) head romaine lettuce, shredded (4 cups)
- 1 (15-ounce) can chickpeas, rinsed and drained
- 4 ounces reduced-fat feta cheese, crumbled (¾ cup)
- 4 sun-dried tomatoes packed in oil, thinly sliced, plus 2 tablespoons oil from jar
- 2 tablespoons fresh lemon juice
- Salt and freshly ground black pepper

Season tofu with salt and pepper. Coat a large nonstick skillet with cooking spray and heat over medium-high heat. Add tofu and cook until browned, 2 to 3 minutes per side. Transfer to a cutting board.

Combine lettuce, chickpeas, feta, tomatoes, oil from tomatoes, and lemon juice in a large mixing bowl. Cut tofu into bite-size pieces, add to lettuce mixture, and toss to combine. Season with salt and pepper to taste and serve.

Makes 4 (2-cup) servings

NUTRITION AT A GLANCE

Per serving: 260 calories, 13 g fat, 3.5 g saturated fat, 19 g protein, 20 g carbohydrate, 5 g dietary fiber, 760 mg sodium

Veggie Burrito

PREP TIME: 5 minutes   **COOK TIME:** 25 minutes

Nutty and satisfying, protein-rich kasha makes an innovative appearance in this delicious veggie burrito. If you want to increase the heat, use spicy salsa in place of medium.

1 tablespoon extra virgin olive oil

1 small onion, chopped

½ cup kasha

1 cup water

4 (8-inch) whole-wheat tortillas

1 (15-ounce) can kidney beans, rinsed and drained

½ head iceberg lettuce, shredded (4 cups)

1 cup refrigerated fresh salsa

2 ounces shredded reduced-fat cheddar cheese (½ cup)

Salt and freshly ground black pepper

Heat oil in a medium saucepan over medium heat. Add onion and cook until softened, about 5 minutes. Add kasha and cook 2 minutes more, stirring constantly. Add water, cover, and cook until water is absorbed, 10 to 12 minutes.

When kasha has almost finished cooking, warm tortillas in the oven or microwave according to package directions. Cover with foil to keep warm.

Add beans with liquid to cooked kasha, stir, and cook until beans are heated through, about 2 minutes. Season mixture to taste with salt and pepper.

Lay tortillas on a flat surface, fill evenly with kasha mixture, and top with lettuce, salsa, and cheese. Fold in the sides of each tortilla and roll up to form burrito. Serve seam side down.

Makes 4 servings

NUTRITION AT A GLANCE

Per serving: 390 calories, 11 g fat, 2.5 g saturated fat, 15 g protein, 57 g carbohydrate, 8 g dietary fiber, 730 mg sodium

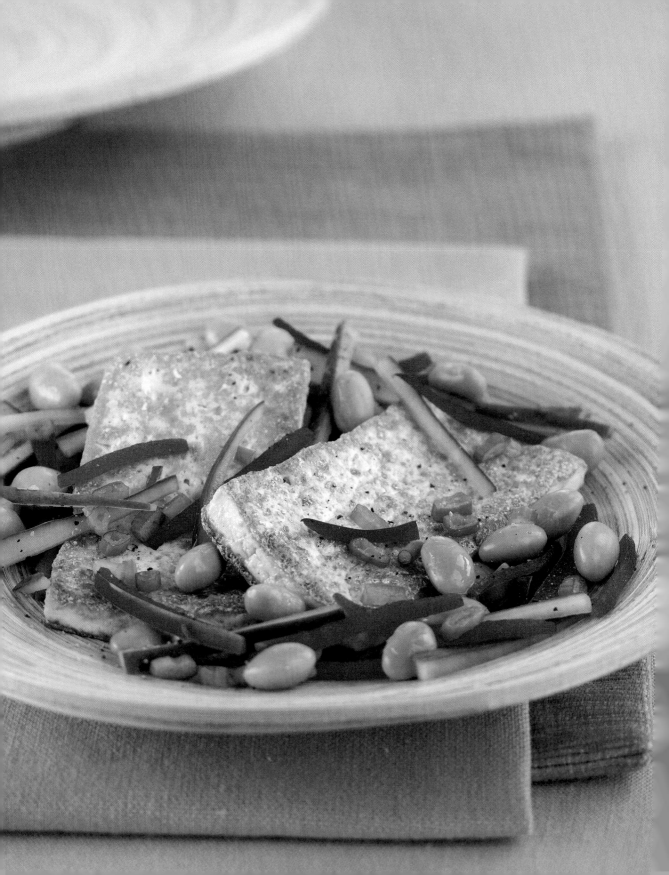

Gingered Tofu Salad

PREP TIME: 15 minutes   **COOK TIME:** 15 minutes

This colorful combination of crisp vegetables and warm tofu makes a quick and tasty protein-packed meal. Make sure to press most of the liquid out of the tofu so that it browns well when seared. Look for edamame (Japanese soybeans) in the frozen section of your supermarket.

2 cups frozen shelled edamame beans

1 (15-ounce) package extra-firm tofu

2 tablespoons finely minced fresh ginger

1 tablespoon canola oil

2 medium cucumbers, peeled, seeded, and thinly sliced

1 medium red bell pepper, thinly sliced

2 scallions, thinly sliced

1 tablespoon dark sesame oil

1 tablespoon low-sodium soy sauce

Salt and freshly ground black pepper

Bring a medium saucepan of salted water to a boil. Add edamame and cook 5 minutes. Drain.

Slice tofu into 8 (½-inch) slices. Lay flat on paper towels, top with another layer of paper towels, and gently press out liquid. Rub with ginger and season well with salt and pepper.

Heat canola oil in a large skillet over medium-high heat. Brown tofu on both sides until lightly golden, 2 to 3 minutes per side. Remove from heat.

Combine edamame, cucumbers, bell pepper, scallions, sesame oil, and soy sauce in a mixing bowl. Season to taste with salt and pepper. Divide salad among 4 plates, top with tofu, and serve.

Makes 4 servings

NUTRITION AT A GLANCE

Per serving: 310 calories, 17 g fat, 2 g saturated fat, 22 g protein, 18 g carbohydrate, 8 g dietary fiber, 200 mg sodium

Soupe au Pistou

PREP TIME: 5 minutes   **COOK TIME: 30 minutes**

Pistou refers to a French basil sauce and is the stuff that makes this soup really shine. Use a simple store-bought pesto and in just over 30 minutes you'll have a hearty, high-protein soup that seems fancy but couldn't be easier to prepare. You can enjoy this soup in phase 1 if you skip the pasta; just remember that the protein level will drop, so eat it as an appetizer and not an entrée.

- 1 teaspoon extra-virgin olive oil
- 1 small onion, diced
- 1 small zucchini, chopped
- 2 garlic cloves, minced
- 3 cups vegetable broth plus 1 cup water
- 1 cup canned crushed tomatoes
- 2 cups frozen shelled edamame beans, thawed
- 4 ounces spelt or whole-wheat elbows, cooked al dente (1 to 2 minutes less than package directions indicate)
- 8 teaspoons pesto (from a jar)
- Salt and freshly ground black pepper

Heat oil in a heavy-bottomed saucepan over medium heat. Add onion and cook until softened, about 5 minutes. Add zucchini and garlic; cook 2 minutes more.

Add broth, water, tomatoes, and edamame. Bring to a low boil. Reduce heat; simmer until beans are tender, about 20 minutes. Add pasta and cook until heated through, about 1 minute. Season with salt and pepper to taste. Ladle into bowls, drizzle with pesto, and serve.

Makes 4 (2-cup) entrée servings or 8 (1-cup) appetizer servings

NUTRITION AT A GLANCE

Per serving: 300 calories, 13 g fat, 2 g saturated fat, 16 g protein, 32 g carbohydrate, 5 g dietary fiber, 540 mg sodium

Portobello Burgers

PREP TIME: 20 minutes   **COOK TIME: 25 minutes**

Meaty mushrooms—combined with protein-packed textured vegetable protein (TVP), provolone cheese, and sun-dried tomatoes—make these vegetarian burgers hearty and super flavorful. TVP is a favorite vegetarian source of nonanimal protein and can be found at health food stores. If you have extra time, form the burgers ahead and refrigerate for 30 minutes for easier handling.

1 cup textured vegetable protein (TVP)

4 ounces provolone cheese, shredded (1 cup)

1 large egg, lightly beaten

3 tablespoons extra-virgin olive oil, divided

2 garlic cloves, minced

3 medium portobello mushrooms, stemmed and chopped

1 small onion, finely chopped

1 small zucchini, coarsely grated

¼ cup sun-dried tomatoes (packed in oil), drained and chopped

Salt and freshly ground black pepper

Combine TVP, cheese, egg, ¾ teaspoon salt, and ¼ teaspoon pepper in a mixing bowl; stir to mix well.

Heat 2 tablespoons of the oil in a large nonstick skillet over medium-high heat. Add garlic and sauté until fragrant, 30 seconds. Add mushrooms, onion, and zucchini; sauté, stirring often, until vegetables are softened and liquid is evaporated, 8 minutes. Stir in tomatoes.

Add vegetable mixture to egg mixture; stir to mix well. Cover and let stand 5 minutes.

Shape vegetable mixture into 6 (3-inch) patties. Heat remaining oil in a clean skillet over medium heat. Cook patties, turning once with a wide spatula, until lightly browned, 3 minutes per side.

Makes 6 servings

NUTRITION AT A GLANCE

Per serving: 230 calories, 16 g fat, 5 g saturated fat, 14 g protein, 11 g carbohydrate, 4 g dietary fiber, 190 mg sodium

Hearty Miso Soup with Soba

PREP TIME: 10 minutes   COOK TIME: 10 minutes

Miso paste (made from soybeans) and soba noodles (made with buckwheat flour) are flavorful, protein-rich Japanese staples that can be found in the Asian section of supermarkets and most health food stores. We suggest using white mushrooms, but you can also try shiitakes or any other favorite. Since miso is naturally salty, you won't need extra salt to season this dish.

- 4 cups water
- ¼ cup miso paste
- 4 ounces white mushrooms, sliced
- 4 ounces soba noodles
- 1 (12.3-ounce) package silken firm tofu, diced
- 4 ounces baby spinach (5 to 6 cups)
- 3 scallions, thinly sliced diagonally
- Freshly ground black pepper

Bring water to a boil in a large saucepan; reduce to a simmer and stir in miso paste. Add mushrooms and noodles and cook for 5 minutes. Add tofu, spinach, and scallions; cook until heated through, about 1 minute. Season with pepper to taste and serve hot.

Makes 4 (1¾-cup) servings

NUTRITION AT A GLANCE

Per serving: 200 calories, 3.5 g fat, 0 g saturated fat, 14 g protein, 32 g carbohydrate, 3 g dietary fiber, 1060 mg sodium

Cauliflower and Kale Bake

PREP TIME: 25 minutes   **COOK TIME:** 35 minutes

Cauliflower and kale become tender and buttery when baked in a flavorful broth, as they are in this eggless casserole-style dish. A cheesy tofu topping adds enough protein to make it a hearty vegetarian supper. Serve quarter portions as a side to any dish.

- 1 tablespoon extra-virgin olive oil, divided
- 2 onions, thinly sliced
- 1 bunch kale (1¼ pounds), tough stems removed and leaves coarsely chopped (10 cups)
- ¾ cup vegetable broth
- 3 pounds cauliflower, cut into florets (8 cups)
- 8 ounces firm tofu, crumbled
- 1 cup shredded reduced-fat sharp cheddar cheese
- 1 cup Italian-flavored whole-wheat bread crumbs
- 3 garlic cloves, minced

 Salt and freshly ground black pepper

Heat oven to 350°F. Lightly coat a 9- by 13-inch baking dish with cooking spray.

    Heat 1 tablespoon of the oil in a large straight-sided skillet over medium-high heat. Add onions and cook 2 minutes; reduce heat to medium. Add kale and broth;

cover and cook, stirring occasionally, until kale is almost tender, about 5 minutes.

Add cauliflower, cover, and cook, stirring occasionally, until cauliflower is crisp-tender, about 8 minutes. Season with salt and pepper to taste and transfer mixture to baking dish.

Combine tofu, cheese, bread crumbs, garlic, ¼ teaspoon salt, and ¼ teaspoon pepper in a bowl; stir to mix well. Spoon evenly over the vegetables. Bake, uncovered, until cheese melts, about 20 minutes. Let stand 5 minutes before serving.

Makes 6 servings

NUTRITION AT A GLANCE

Per serving: 300 calories, 15 g fat, 7 g saturated fat, 22 g protein, 28 g carbohydrate, 7 g dietary fiber, 260 mg sodium

Italian-Style Tofu Bake

PREP TIME: 10 minutes   **COOK TIME:** 20 minutes

This cheesy baked dish, packed with spinach and flavored with tasty sun-dried tomatoes, is a great alternative to traditional pizza.

> 2 teaspoons extra-virgin olive oil
>
> 2 garlic cloves, minced
>
> 10 ounces fresh spinach, thick stems trimmed (5 cups packed or 10 cups loosely packed)
>
> 1 (15-ounce) package firm tofu, sliced lengthwise into 8 pieces
>
> 1 tablespoon dried basil, divided
>
> 4 sun-dried tomatoes (packed in oil), drained and thinly sliced
>
> ½ cup shredded part-skim mozzarella cheese
>
> 2 tablespoons freshly grated Parmesan cheese
>
> Salt and freshly ground black pepper

Heat oven to 400°F.

Heat oil over medium heat in a large skillet. Add garlic and cook until softened, about 1 minute. Add spinach, cover, and cook until wilted and tender, about 3 minutes; season with salt and pepper. Remove from heat.

Lay tofu slices in a single layer in a 9- by 13-inch baking dish. Sprinkle each slice with a pinch of the basil.

Top tofu slices evenly with spinach, tomatoes, mozzarella, Parmesan, and remaining basil. Bake until tofu is hot and cheeses are melted and bubbling, about 15 minutes.

Makes 4 servings

NUTRITION AT A GLANCE

Per serving: 190 calories, 12 g fat, 3.5 g saturated fat, 19 g protein, 6 g carbohydrate, 3 g dietary fiber, 280 mg sodium

Tempeh Tacos

PREP TIME: 10 minutes   **COOK TIME:** 11 minutes

Filling these soft tacos with all the goodies makes for a fun and tasty meal. Choose mild, medium, or hot salsa to suit your taste.

    4 (8-inch) low-fat whole-wheat tortillas, quartered

    2 tablespoons extra-virgin olive oil

 1½ (8-ounce) packages tempeh, crumbled

    1 small head iceberg lettuce, shredded

    1 avocado, pitted, peeled, and cut into ¼-inch cubes

  ¾ cup salsa

    2 ounces shredded reduced-fat cheddar cheese (½ cup)

      Salt and freshly ground black pepper

Heat oven to 225°F, lay tortilla pieces on a baking sheet, and heat until warmed through, about 5 minutes (or heat in a microwave according to package directions). Cover with foil to keep warm.

Heat oil in a large nonstick skillet over medium-high heat. Add tempeh and cook until browned and heated through, about 6 minutes. Season with salt and pepper to taste.

Serve tortilla pieces with warm tempeh, lettuce, avocado, salsa, and cheese, letting diners fill their own tacos.

Makes 4 servings

NUTRITION AT A GLANCE

Per serving: 460 calories, 28 g fat, 6 g saturated fat, 27 g protein, 30 g carbohydrate, 7 g dietary fiber, 660 mg sodium

Whole-Wheat Penne with Eggplant and Ricotta

PREP TIME: 15 minutes   **COOK TIME:** 25 minutes

Tossing hot pasta with ricotta cheese creates a quick creamy sauce that's rich in taste and low in fat. Top this dish with fresh parsley or basil, if you have some on hand.

2 tablespoons extra-virgin olive oil, plus more for pan

1½ pounds eggplant, cut into 1-inch cubes

8 ounces whole-wheat or spelt penne

1 small onion, thinly sliced

3 garlic cloves, minced

1 (14.5-ounce) can chopped tomatoes

2 teaspoons balsamic vinegar

1 cup part-skim ricotta cheese

Salt and freshly ground black pepper

Heat oven to 450°F.

Lightly coat a baking pan with oil. Place eggplant in the pan, drizzle with 1 tablespoon of the oil, season with salt and pepper, toss to coat, and spread in an even layer. Bake, stirring once, until eggplant is lightly browned, about 25 minutes.

While eggplant is roasting, cook pasta according to the package directions.

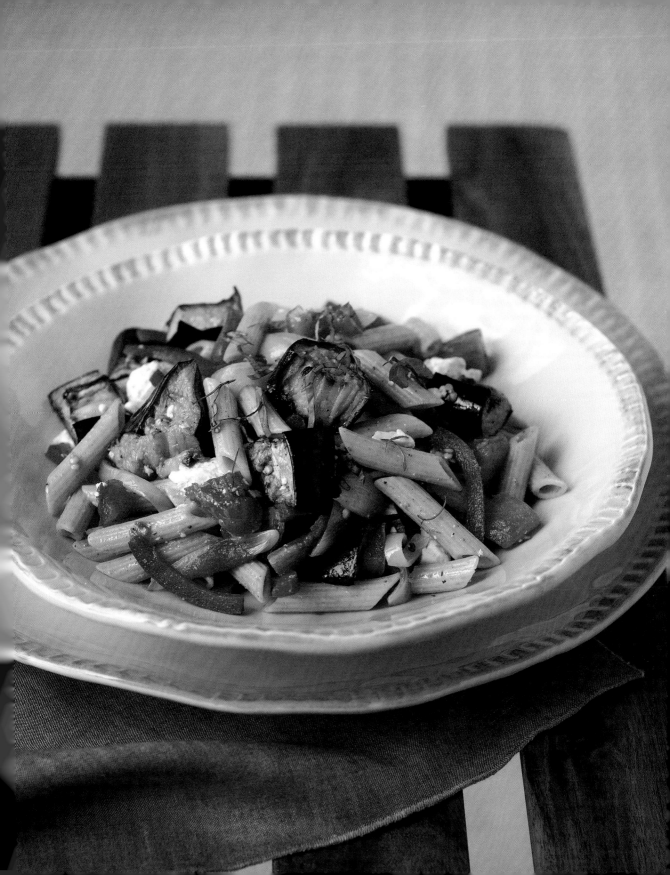

Meanwhile, heat remaining oil in a large skillet over medium-high heat. Add onion and cook, stirring occasionally, until softened, about 5 minutes. Add garlic and cook 1 minute more. Add tomatoes with juice and bring to a boil. Reduce heat to medium-low, cover, and simmer for 3 minutes. Stir in vinegar and season to taste with salt and pepper.

Drain pasta, place in a large bowl, and add tomato mixture, eggplant, and cheese. Toss to combine, season with salt and pepper, and serve.

Makes 4 (2-cup) servings

NUTRITION AT A GLANCE

Per serving: 420 calories, 14 g fat, 4 g saturated fat, 18 g protein, 62 g carbohydrate, 12 g dietary fiber, 320 mg sodium

Quick Bean Chili

PREP TIME: 10 minutes   **COOK TIME:** 25 minutes

Black soybeans and textured vegetable protein (TVP), found in most health food stores, turn this richly flavored vegetarian chili into a high-protein meal. Chipotle peppers add a delightfully smoky and slightly sweet taste, and green tops from scallions offer a dose of beta-carotene.

1 tablespoon extra-virgin olive oil

5 scallions, chopped

1 bell pepper, any color, chopped

1 small zucchini, cut into ½-inch dice

1 (15-ounce) can black soybeans, liquid reserved

1 (15-ounce) can crushed tomatoes

1 canned chipotle chile in adobo, minced, plus 2 tablespoons sauce from can

½ cup textured vegetable protein (TVP)

¼ cup shredded reduced-fat cheddar cheese

Salt and freshly ground black pepper

Heat oil in large saucepan over medium-high heat. Add scallions, bell pepper, and zucchini; cook, stirring occasionally, until vegetables soften, about 5 minutes. Add beans and their liquid, tomatoes, chile, adobo sauce, and TVP. Bring to a low boil, reduce to a simmer, cover, and cook 20 minutes. Season to taste with salt and pepper. Ladle into bowls and serve with cheese.

Makes 4 (generous 1-cup) servings

NUTRITION AT A GLANCE

Per serving: 190 calories, 6 g fat, 1.5 g saturated fat, 15 g protein, 20 g carbohydrate, 8 g dietary fiber, 260 mg sodium

Tempeh Stir-Fry

PREP TIME: 10 minutes   **COOK TIME: 12 minutes**

Peanut butter is the surprise ingredient in the sauce for this quick vegetarian dish. It creates a smooth and nutty background for tasty veggies and tempeh. Look for tempeh (a pressed soybean cake) and rice vinegar in health food and Asian markets; rice vinegar can also be found in most supermarkets.

¼ cup creamy trans-fat-free peanut butter

3 tablespoons low-sodium soy sauce, divided

2 tablespoons rice vinegar

1 tablespoon canola oil, divided

2 (8-ounce) packages soy tempeh, cut into 1-inch pieces

4 garlic cloves, minced

1 pound white mushrooms, sliced

1 bunch scallions, cut into 1-inch pieces

2 red bell peppers, cut into thin strips

Whisk together peanut butter, 2 tablespoons of the soy sauce, and vinegar in a small bowl until smooth.

Heat ½ tablespoon of the oil in a large nonstick skillet or wok over high heat. Add tempeh and cook, stirring frequently, until golden, about 4 minutes. Add remaining soy sauce and toss to coat. Transfer tempeh to a plate.

Heat remaining oil in the same skillet over medium-high heat; add garlic and cook 30 seconds. Add mushrooms, scallions, and bell peppers; cook until the vegetables are crisp-tender, about 4 minutes. Add tempeh and peanut butter mixture, toss until all ingredients are well coated, and serve.

Makes 4 (2-cup) servings

NUTRITION AT A GLANCE

Per serving: 370 calories, 18 g fat, 4 g saturated fat, 32 g protein, 24 g carbohydrate, 10 g dietary fiber, 500 mg sodium

Lentil and Kale Stew

PREP TIME: 10 minutes   **COOK TIME: 30 minutes**

This is so hearty that calling it a mere soup just didn't seem right! It's jam-packed with protein and rich earthy flavor.

1 tablespoon extra-virgin olive oil

4 celery stalks, finely chopped

1 small onion, chopped

2 garlic cloves, minced

2 (15-ounce) cans brown lentils, rinsed and drained

1 cup canned crushed tomatoes

3 cups low-sodium tomato vegetable juice

1 (½-pound) bunch kale, tough stems removed and leaves roughly chopped (5 to 6 cups)

1 cup shredded reduced-fat cheddar cheese

Salt and freshly ground black pepper

Heat oil in a large saucepan over medium-high heat. Add celery, onion, and garlic; cook 5 minutes, stirring occasionally (do not brown).

Add lentils, tomatoes, juice, and kale; stir to combine and bring to a simmer. Reduce heat to low, cover, and cook 15 to 20 minutes. Season to taste with salt and pepper. Ladle into bowls, top with cheese, and serve.

Makes 4 (2-cup) servings

NUTRITION AT A GLANCE

Per serving: 280 calories, 10 g fat, 4.5 g saturated fat, 17 g protein, 31 g carbohydrate, 7 g dietary fiber, 600 mg sodium

Spelt Pasta with Chickpeas and Broccoli

PREP TIME: 10 minutes   **COOK TIME:** 20 minutes

High in fiber, protein, and B vitamins, spelt (an ancient cousin of wheat) is full of nutty flavor. Look for it in health food stores and in the health food section of some supermarkets or use whole-wheat pasta instead.

- 1 (¾-pound) head broccoli, cut into florets (2 to 3 cups)
- 8 ounces spelt or whole-wheat linguine
- 1 tablespoon extra-virgin olive oil
- 1 onion, diced
- 2 garlic cloves, minced
- 1 (15-ounce) can chickpeas, rinsed and drained
- 1 tablespoon fresh lemon juice
- ¼ cup finely grated Parmesan cheese (optional)
- Salt and freshly ground black pepper

Blanch broccoli in a large saucepan of salted boiling water until crisp-tender, about 3 minutes. Remove from water with a slotted spoon and set aside. Add pasta to water and cook according to package directions. Scoop out ½ cup of pasta cooking liquid and reserve. Drain pasta.

Heat oil in a large skillet over medium heat. Add onion and garlic and cook, stirring occasionally, until softened, about 3 minutes. Add chickpeas, broccoli, and pasta cooking liquid. Bring to a simmer and cook until heated through, about 2 minutes. Add pasta and lemon juice; stir to coat.

Cook until water is mostly evaporated, about 3 more minutes. Season with salt and pepper to taste and serve with cheese, if using.

Makes 4 (1½-cup) servings

NUTRITION AT A GLANCE

Per serving: 340 calories, 6 g fat, ½ g saturated fat, 14 g protein, 64 g carbohydrate, 10 g dietary fiber, 320 mg sodium

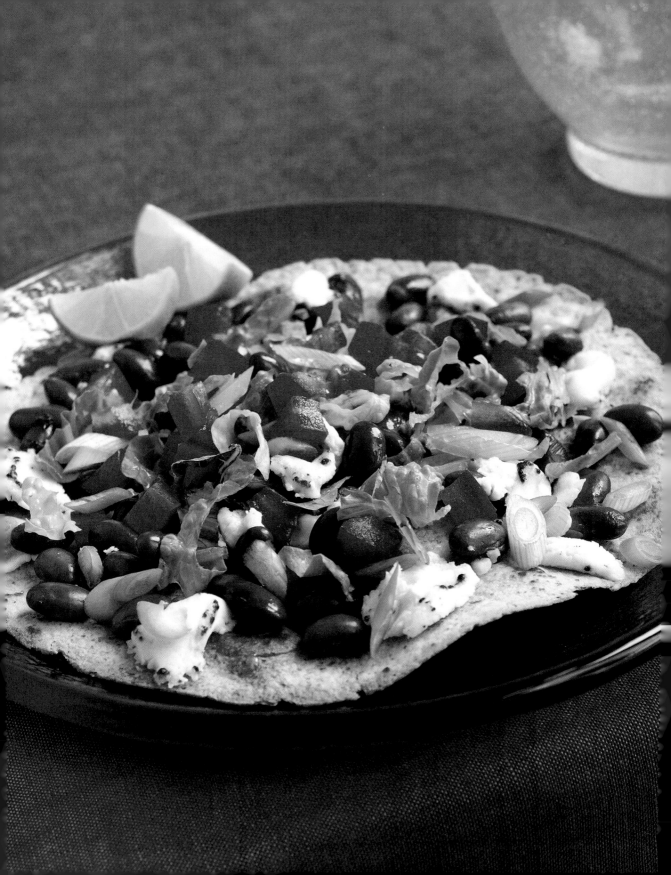

Black Bean and Goat Cheese Tostadas

PREP TIME: 10 minutes   **COOK TIME:** 20 minutes

A fresh squeeze of lime gives a tasty, tart balance to garlicky beans in this Mexican-inspired dish. Black soybeans are packed with protein and are available in most health food markets. If you can't find them, use regular black beans.

- 4 (8-inch) whole-wheat tortillas
- 2 teaspoons extra-virgin olive oil
- 1 large garlic clove, minced
- 1 (15-ounce) can black soybeans, rinsed and drained
- 4 ounces reduced-fat goat cheese, crumbled (¾ cup)
- ½ (1-pound) head romaine lettuce, chopped (4 cups)
- 2 medium tomatoes, diced
- 3 scallions, thinly sliced
- 1 lime, quartered
- Salt and freshly ground black pepper

Heat oven to 400°F.

Lightly spray tortillas with cooking spray and place, slightly overlapping, on a baking sheet. Bake until lightly puffed and browned, about 10 minutes. Set aside to cool.

While tortillas are toasting, heat oil in a medium saucepan over medium heat. Add garlic and cook until softened, about 1 minute. Stir in beans and heat until warmed through. Season with salt and pepper and remove from heat.

With tortillas still on the baking sheet, top with beans and cheese; bake until cheese is melted, about 5 minutes. Remove from the oven and top with lettuce, tomatoes, and scallions. Squeeze lime over top and serve hot.

Makes 4 servings

NUTRITION AT A GLANCE

Per serving: 290 calories, 10 g fat, 2.5 g saturated fat, 13 g protein, 35 g carbohydrate, 7 g dietary fiber, 380 mg sodium

Eggplant Bulgur Lasagna

PREP TIME: 25 minutes   **COOK TIME: 35 minutes**

Spend some extra time making a batch or two of this delicious veggie dish. Then freeze indivdual portions, which can be thawed and reheated in the microwave in minutes when you're ready to eat.

- 1 medium eggplant
- 2 teaspoons extra-virgin olive oil
- 1 small onion, diced
- 2 garlic cloves, minced
- 1 cup bulgur wheat
- 1½ teaspoons dried oregano
- 1 (14-ounce) package extra-firm tofu, cut into bite-size cubes
- 1½ cups low-sugar tomato sauce (from a jar)
- 1½ cups shredded reduced-fat mozzarella cheese
- Salt and freshly ground black pepper

Heat oven to 450°F. Line 2 baking sheets with foil.

Slice eggplant lengthwise into 12 slices and spray both sides with cooking spray. Place in a single layer on baking sheets and season with salt and pepper. Bake until lightly browned, about 15 minutes.

While eggplant is baking, heat oil in a medium saucepan over medium heat. Add onion and cook until softened, about 3 minutes. Add garlic, bulgur, and oregano; cook for about 2 minutes. Stir in tofu and 1½ cups water and bring to a simmer; cover and cook until water has been absorbed, about 15 minutes. Season with salt and pepper.

Spread ½ cup sauce in an 11- by 17-inch baking dish. Cover with a single layer of eggplant slices. Top with 2 cups bulgur mixture and an additional ½ cup of tomato sauce. Repeat with another layer of eggplant slices and bulgur. Top with remaining eggplant slices, remaining sauce, and cheese. Bake until cheese is lightly browned and melted, about 20 minutes. Serve hot.

Makes 6 servings

NUTRITION AT A GLANCE

Per serving: 260 calories, 8 g fat, 3 g saturated fat, 17 g protein, 27 g carbohydrate, 9 g dietary fiber, 410 mg sodium

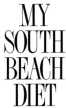

MY SOUTH BEACH DIET

"The South Beach Diet lifestyle is so realistic. If you fall off-track, you can always get back on."

As a competitive figure skater, I always paid strict attention to my weight. While on the ice, I needed to look good and have enough energy to sustain a heart-pumping performance. Luckily, I had always been naturally slender and even managed to maintain my weight after I decided to stop touring and training so rigorously. But once I became pregnant with twins 10 years ago, I found it hard to take off the post-pregnancy weight. As with most moms I know, I had less time for working out.

I'll admit I was rather lazy about finding the right eating plan until my skating partner, Ken Shelley, and I were invited to appear in "Legends on Ice," taking place in November 2004 in California. I knew I had to get rid of the extra pounds if I wanted to dazzle on the rink.

I went straight to the healthy eating book section at my local natural food store, hoping to find more information on meal plans to try. As I flipped through the various diet books, my 8-year-old son kept pointing to *The South Beach Diet.* I had heard a little about the South Beach Diet and assumed it was more of a fad than a realistic option. My little boy finally wore me down, and I ended up leaving the store with Dr. Agatston's program in hand.

As soon as I opened The South Beach Diet, I knew it was the right choice and definitely not a passing trend. And the fact that Dr. Agatston was a respected cardiologist made me feel safe. My husband and I began this lifestyle together in July 2004, and over the course of a couple of months, I lost 15 pounds and my husband lost 12 pounds. The things that kept me the most interested were the recipes. I loved the Poached Salmon with Cucumber-Dill Sauce, the breakfast quiches, and the Spinach-Stuffed Mushrooms. I also loved the fact that I could have wine, reduced-fat cheese, and nuts. Sometimes my husband would come home and ask, "Aren't we on a diet?" because the food did not look like typical "diet" food. Everything was just so delicious.

When the time came for "Legends on Ice," I felt I looked my best. I am just so grateful for the South Beach Diet. It's so easy, delicious, and healthy. Thank you, Dr. Agatston!

JOJO STARBUCK, MADISON, NEW JERSEY
TWO-TIME OLYMPIAN AND WORLD BRONZE MEDALIST,
PAIRS FIGURE SKATING

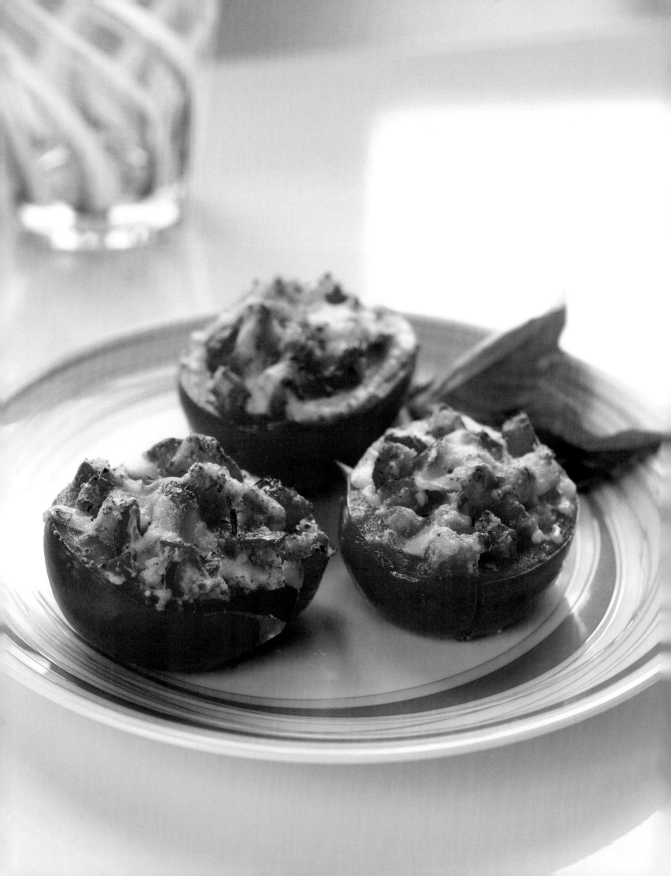

SIDES

Humble though it may seem, a good side dish can make the meal. In fact, here's a great tip you can use anytime: A 15-minute side paired with a simple piece of grilled chicken, meat, or fish is the perfect solution for a time-tight weeknight meal. Put leftovers into a sealed baggie and the next day's lunch is practically covered.

"Good carb" sides, made with low-fat foods such as quinoa and brown rice, abound in the coming pages, alongside updated classics, like Sesame Green Beans, Baked Sweet Potato Fries, Roasted Spicy Cauliflower, Ratatouille, and Sauteed Mushrooms with Thyme. Vegetables that might be unfamiliar, like fiber-rich broccoli rabe (an excellent source of B vitamins and cancer-fighting phytochemicals), tasty escarole, celery root, and turnips are likely to become new favorites.

◄ *Stuffed Baked Tomatoes (page 414)*

413

Stuffed Baked Tomatoes

PREP TIME: 10 minutes   **COOK TIME:** 10 minutes

This warm, cheesy side dish pairs tomato and basil with mozzarella and Parmesan cheese—a match made in heaven if there ever was one! Serve it with grilled chicken, steak, or fish.

4 plum tomatoes, halved lengthwise

3 ounces shredded part-skim mozzarella cheese (½ cup)

¼ cup roughly chopped fresh basil leaves

2 tablespoons freshly grated Parmesan cheese

1 garlic clove, minced

Salt and freshly ground black pepper

Heat oven to 400°F.

Scoop out the inside of each tomato half with a melon baller and roughly chop the scooped pulp. Combine tomato pulp, mozzarella, basil, Parmesan, garlic, and a pinch of salt and pepper.

Place tomatoes, cut side up, on a baking sheet. Spoon in tomato mixture and bake until cheese is melted and lightly browned, about 10 minutes. Serve warm.

Makes 4 servings

NUTRITION AT A GLANCE

Per serving: 90 calories, 5 g fat, 3 g saturated fat, 7 g protein, 4 g carbohydrate, 0 g dietary fiber, 230 mg sodium

Roasted Spicy Cauliflower

PREP TIME: 5 minutes   **COOK TIME:** 30 minutes

You're in for a treat with this recipe because roasting cauliflower makes it so tender that it melts in your mouth. This simple method turns the firm, white florets into delicate, golden brown, slightly sweet morsels—a delightful and delectable change of pace.

> 1 (2- to 2½-pound) head cauliflower, cored and cut into florets (4 to 6 cups)
>
> 2 tablespoons extra-virgin olive oil
>
> 1 teaspoon red pepper flakes
>
> ¼ teaspoon salt
>
> ¼ teaspoon freshly ground black pepper

Heat oven to 400°F.

Place cauliflower, oil, red pepper flakes, salt, and pepper in a mixing bowl; toss to combine. Arrange in a single layer on a heavy-bottomed baking sheet or in a large baking dish. Roast until softened and golden brown, 25 to 30 minutes.

Makes 4 (2-cup) servings

NUTRITION AT A GLANCE

Per serving: 110 calories, 7 g fat, 1.5 g saturated fat, 4 g protein, 11 g carbohydrate, 5 g dietary fiber, 210 mg sodium

Sesame Green Beans

PREP TIME: 10 minutes   COOK TIME: 5 minutes

Sesame oil gives body and nuttiness to these crisp garlicky beans. This simple and very pretty salad can be made up to 12 hours in advance and is great for a no-fuss weeknight meal. Try it alongside grilled steak or chicken. Leftovers, if there are any, will be even more flavorful the next day.

      1 tablespoon plus 2 teaspoons low-sodium soy
          sauce

     ¾ teaspoon dark sesame oil

      1 small garlic clove, minced

      1 pound green beans, trimmed

    12 cherry tomatoes, halved

          Salt

Whisk together soy sauce, oil, and garlic in a large mixing bowl.

Bring a saucepan of salted water to a boil. Add beans and cook until tender, about 2 minutes. Drain and run under cold water for 30 seconds. Add beans and tomatoes to soy sauce mixture and toss to combine. Serve at room temperature or refrigerate until ready to serve.

Makes 4 servings

NUTRITION AT A GLANCE

Per serving: 50 calories, 1 g fat, 0 g saturated fat, 2 g protein, 8 g carbohydrate, 4 g dietary fiber, 220 mg sodium

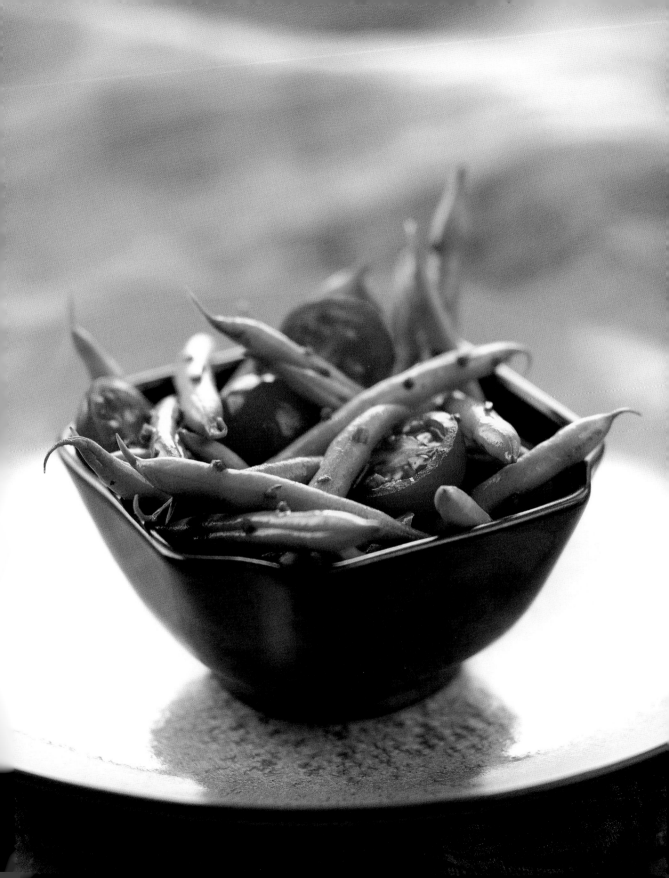

Quinoa Pilaf

PREP TIME: 5 minutes　　　**COOK TIME: 20 minutes**

Both first-time and well-seasoned quinoa eaters will love this dish. In addition to being delicious, quinoa is an excellent source of plant protein and also provides iron, vitamin E, and fiber.

1¾ cups water

¾ cup quinoa

½ cup shelled unsalted pistachios

1 tablespoon plus 1 teaspoon extra-virgin olive oil, divided

1 small red bell pepper, finely diced

2 scallions, thinly sliced

2 teaspoons white wine vinegar

Salt and freshly ground black pepper

Heat oven or toaster oven to 350°F.

Combine water and quinoa in a medium saucepan; bring to a boil. Reduce heat, cover, and simmer until tender, about 15 minutes. Drain and place in a mixing bowl.

While quinoa is cooking, spread pistachios on a baking tray and bake until lightly browned and fragrant, about 10 minutes. Cool and roughly chop.

Heat 1 teaspoon of the oil in a small nonstick skillet over medium heat. Add bell pepper and scallions and cook until softened, about 3 minutes. Add to quinoa, along with pistachios, vinegar, and remaining oil; stir to combine. Season with salt and pepper to taste and serve.

Makes 4 (¾-cup) servings

NUTRITION AT A GLANCE

Per serving: 260 calories, 14 g fat, 1.5 g saturated fat, 8 g protein, 28 g carbohydrate, 4 g dietary fiber, 85 mg sodium

Chinese-Style Broccoli

PREP TIME: 10 minutes   **COOK TIME:** 8 minutes

Ordinary broccoli springs to life with this garlicky lemon-soy dressing. Serve it with any Asian-flavored dish or even a simple grilled chicken or shrimp skewer.

- 1 tablespoon plus 1 teaspoon canola oil
- 1 (1½-pound) head broccoli, cut into florets (6 cups)
- 2 tablespoons low-sodium soy sauce
- 2 garlic cloves, minced
- 2 teaspoons fresh lemon juice

Heat oil in a large wok or high-sided skillet over medium-high heat. Add broccoli and stir-fry for 2 minutes. Add soy sauce, garlic, and lemon juice; continue to stir-fry until broccoli is crisp-tender, about 5 minutes. Serve hot.

Makes 4 (1-cup) servings

NUTRITION AT A GLANCE

Per serving: 80 calories, 5 g fat, 0 g saturated fat, 4 g protein, 7 g carbohydrate, 3 g dietary fiber, 300 mg sodium

Nutty Brown Rice

PREP TIME: 10 minutes   **COOK TIME: 30 minutes**

Lightly toasted almonds and chopped parsley turn brown rice into a healthy and delicious companion for chicken, fish, or vegetables. Serve it warm or try it cold at a summer picnic or barbecue with a drizzle of extra-virgin olive oil and a teaspoon of fresh lemon juice mixed in just before serving.

- 2 teaspoons extra-virgin olive oil
- 1 small onion, diced
- ½ cup whole-grain, quick-cooking brown rice (page 14)
- 1 cup vegetable broth or lower-sodium chicken broth
- ⅓ cup water
- ¾ cup sliced almonds
- 2 tablespoons chopped fresh parsley
- Salt and freshly ground black pepper

Heat oven or toaster oven to 350°F.

Heat oil in a medium saucepan over medium-low heat. Add onion, cover, and cook until softened, about 3 minutes. Add rice and stir until well coated. Add broth and water, bring to a simmer, cover, and cook until rice is tender and liquid is absorbed, about 30 minutes.

While rice is cooking, spread almonds on a baking tray. Bake until lightly browned and fragrant, about 5 minutes. Set aside to cool.

Stir almonds into rice and season with salt and pepper to taste. Add parsley just before serving.

Makes 4 (¾-cup) servings

NUTRITION AT A GLANCE

Per serving: 230 calories, 12 g fat, 1 g saturated fat, 7 g protein, 25 g carbohydrate, 3 g dietary fiber, 240 mg sodium

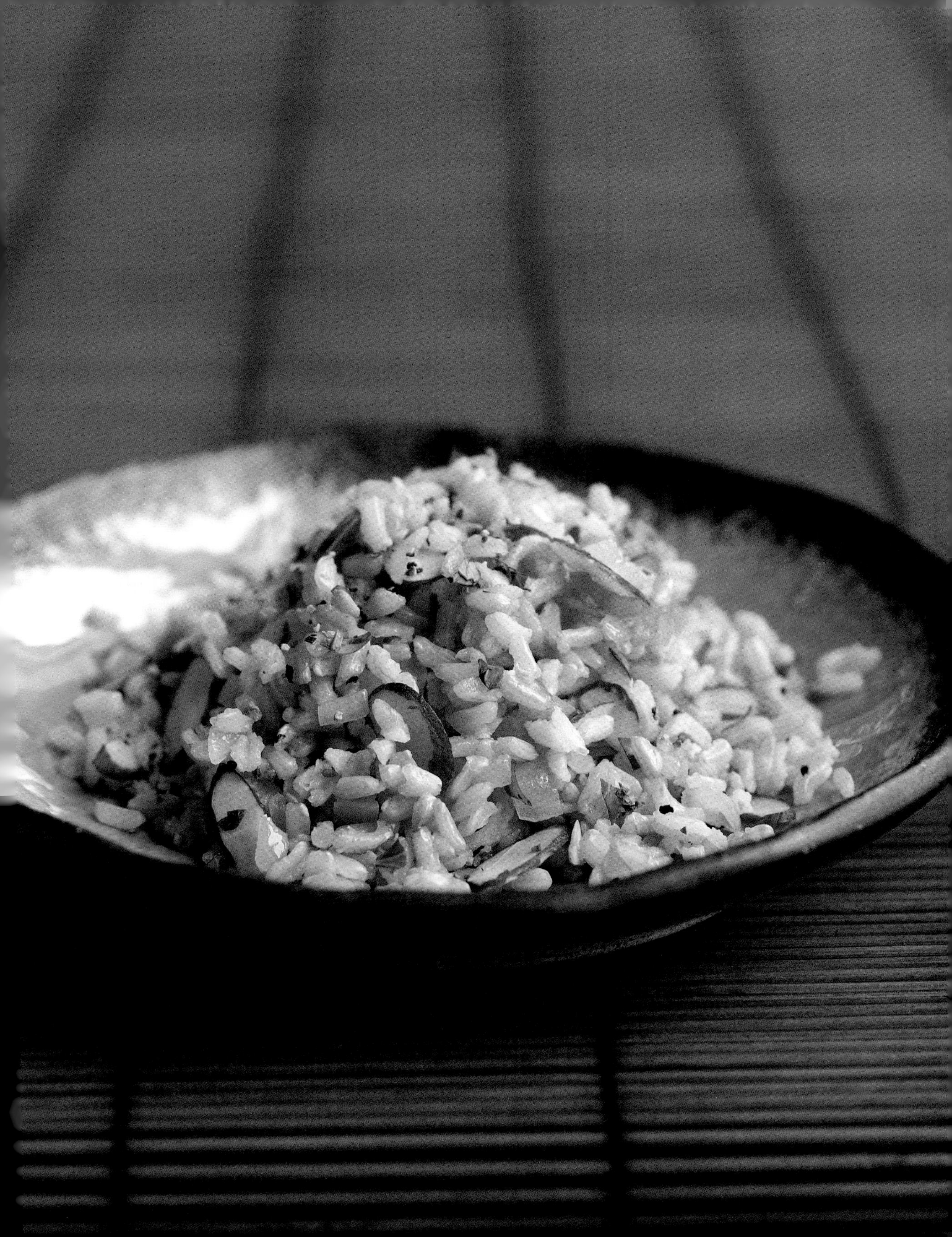

Green Beans with Mushrooms and Balsamic

PREP TIME: 5 minutes   **COOK TIME: 10 minutes**

This delicious combination of warm mushrooms, tender beans, and sweet balsamic vinegar provides ample amounts of fiber, folate, and vitamin C. Pair it with steak or chicken or just eat it solo.

1 pound green beans, trimmed

1 tablespoon extra-virgin olive oil

8 ounces white mushrooms, sliced

1 tablespoon balsamic vinegar

Salt and freshly ground black pepper

Cook green beans in a saucepan of salted boiling water until crisp-tender, about 4 minutes. Drain.

Heat oil in a large skillet over medium-high heat. Add mushrooms and cook until browned, about 5 minutes. Add green beans and vinegar; season to taste with salt and pepper, toss to combine, and serve warm.

Makes 4 servings

NUTRITION AT A GLANCE

Per serving: 80 calories, 3.5 g fat, 0 g saturated fat, 3 g protein, 11 g carbohydrate, 4 g dietary fiber, 75 mg sodium

Sautéed Mushrooms with Thyme

PREP TIME: 5 minutes   **COOK TIME:** 10 minutes

These tasty, aromatic mushrooms are a great match for steak, chicken, or fish. They also make a nice holiday side dish. You can use rosemary, oregano, basil, or a mix of your favorite herbs in place of thyme when you're ready for a change.

    1 tablespoon extra-virgin olive oil
    ½ small red onion, thinly sliced
    ¾ teaspoon dried thyme
    1 pound white or cremini mushrooms, quartered
      Salt and freshly ground black pepper

Heat oil in a large nonstick skillet over medium-high heat. Add onion and thyme, reduce heat to medium, and cook until softened and lightly brown, about 2 minutes.

Add mushrooms and cook, stirring occasionally, until tender and lightly browned, about 8 minutes. Season well with salt and pepper and serve hot.

Makes 4 (generous ½-cup) servings

NUTRITION AT A GLANCE

Per serving: 60 calories, 3.5 g fat, ½ g saturated fat, 3 g protein, 6 g carbohydrate, 0 g dietary fiber, 80 mg sodium

Baked Sweet Potato Fries

PREP TIME: 5 minutes **COOK TIME:** 30 minutes

Sweet potato makes these golden oven fries much healthier than the fried white potatoes we all grew up eating. If you want to add a spicy touch, use Hungarian hot paprika.

  2 medium sweet potatoes, scrubbed and dried

  1 tablespoon extra-virgin olive oil

  ¼ teaspoon salt

  ½ teaspoon paprika

Heat oven to 425°F.

Slice each sweet potato lengthwise into 8 pieces. Toss with oil, salt, and paprika. Spread in a single layer on a baking sheet and bake until lightly browned on the bottom, about 15 minutes.

Turn slices and bake until bottom is browned and potatoes are tender, about 10 minutes more. Serve hot.

Makes 4 servings

NUTRITION AT A GLANCE

Per serving: 100 calories, 3.5 g fat, 0 g saturated fat, 1 g protein, 17 g carbohydrate, 2 g dietary fiber, 170 mg sodium

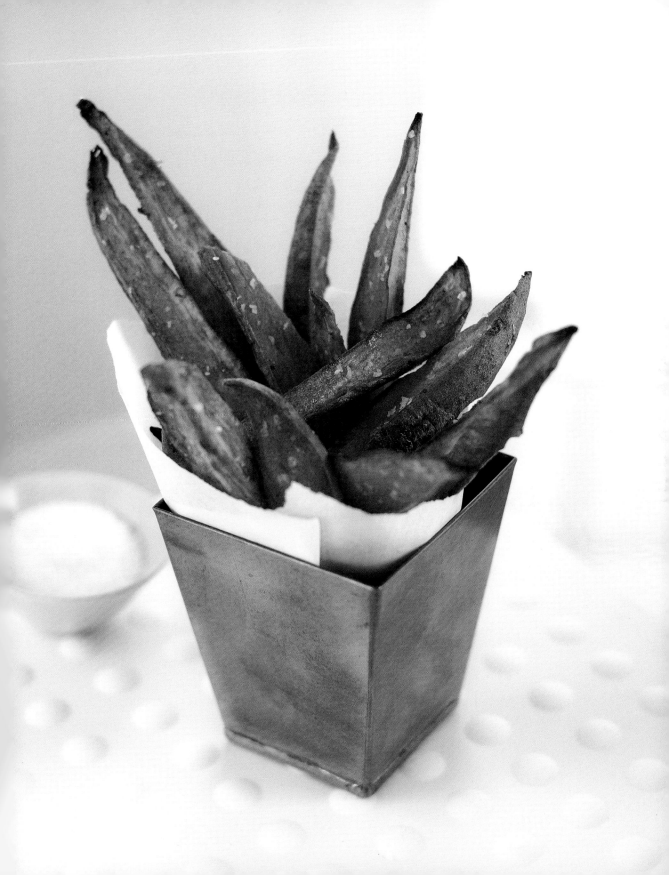

Lemony Sautéed Escarole

PREP TIME: 5 minutes   **COOK TIME:** 10 minutes

Escarole's sturdy leaves become melt-in-your-mouth tender when quickly cooked. Sweet onion and tangy lemon are the perfect foil for its deliciously mild bitterness.

1	tablespoon extra-virgin olive oil
½	small red onion, thinly sliced
2	pounds escarole, halved lengthwise, cored, and cut crosswise into 2-inch strips (15 to 16 cups)
1½	teaspoons fresh lemon juice
	Salt and freshly ground black pepper

Heat oil in a large skillet over medium-high heat. Add onion, reduce heat to medium, and cook until softened and lightly browned, about 3 minutes.

Increase heat to medium-high. Add escarole in batches, tossing each batch with tongs until wilted before adding the next, until all escarole is wilted, about 3 minutes. Remove from heat, stir in lemon juice, and season with salt and pepper to taste. Serve hot.

Makes 4 (1-cup) servings

NUTRITION AT A GLANCE

Per serving: 70 calories, 4 g fat, ½ g saturated fat, 3 g protein, 8 g carbohydrate, 6 g dietary fiber, 120 mg sodium

Broccoli Rabe with Olives

PREP TIME: 10 minutes   **COOK TIME:** 10 minutes

A popular crucifer, broccoli rabe's pleasantly bitter flavor goes well with citrus and naturally salty olives. Add a pinch of red pepper flakes, if you like a kick. Serve with lamb chops, grilled chicken, or steak.

- 1 tablespoon plus 1 teaspoon extra-virgin olive oil
- 2 garlic cloves, sliced
- 2 pounds broccoli rabe, ends trimmed and roughly chopped (8 to 10 cups)
- ¾ cup hot water
- 2 teaspoons grated lemon zest
- ¼ cup pitted, chopped kalamata olives
- 2 tablespoons fresh lemon juice

  Salt and freshly ground black pepper

Heat oil in a large skillet over medium heat. Add garlic and cook until fragrant, 1 to 2 minutes. Add broccoli rabe, water, and lemon zest; cover and cook until broccoli rabe is wilted and stems are tender, about 4 minutes. Remove from heat, stir in olives and lemon juice, season to taste with salt and pepper, and serve.

Makes 4 (1¼-cup) servings

NUTRITION AT A GLANCE

Per serving: 120 calories, 6 g fat, 1 g saturated fat, 7 g protein, 11 g carbohydrate, 0 g dietary fiber, 190 mg sodium

Roasted Eggplant with Lemon and Olive Oil

PREP TIME: 8 minutes   **COOK TIME: 30 minutes**

Eggplant takes on a delicious, slightly smoky flavor when roasted in a hot oven. Sprinkled with fresh lemon juice and salt, this version is a great match for any meat or fish dish; vegetarians can enjoy it with our Portobello Burgers (page 387) or Italian-Style Tofu Bake (page 392).

> 1 large (1¼-pound) eggplant
>
> 2½ tablespoons extra-virgin olive oil, plus extra for the pan
>
> 1 tablespoon fresh lemon juice
>
> Salt and freshly ground black pepper

Heat oven to 400°F.

Trim eggplant and cut in half lengthwise; cut each half into 4 long wedges. Cut each wedge in half widthwise. Brush a heavy-bottomed baking sheet with oil or line with parchment paper.

Place eggplant pieces, skin side down, on the baking sheet. Brush each with oil and sprinkle with salt and pepper. Roast until softened and golden brown, 25 to

30 minutes. Drizzle with lemon juice, season with extra salt and pepper if needed, and serve hot.

Makes 4 servings

NUTRITION AT A GLANCE

Per serving: 110 calories, 9 g fat, 1.5 g saturated fat, 1 g protein, 8 g carbohydrate, 5 g dietary fiber, 75 mg sodium

Indian-Spiced Lentils

PREP TIME: 5 minutes   **COOK TIME: 25 minutes**

Low in fat and high in protein, lentils are a great source of fiber and folate. When cooking lentils (or dried beans or other legumes), remember that the fresher the product, the quicker the cooking time. Dried beans and legumes do lose flavor over time, so buy fresh (some packages have sell-by dates) and keep them rotating in your pantry.

4 teaspoons extra-virgin olive oil

1 medium onion, diced

2 garlic cloves, minced

1 teaspoon curry powder

1 cup dried lentils, picked over and rinsed

1½ cups lower-sodium chicken broth

2 tablespoons chopped fresh parsley

Salt and freshly ground black pepper

Heat oil in a medium saucepan over medium heat. Add onion and sauté until softened, about 3 minutes. Add garlic and cook 1 minute more. Stir in curry powder and lentils. Add broth, bring to a simmer, cover, and cook until tender, about 20 minutes. Season to taste with salt and pepper. Stir in parsley just before serving.

Makes 4 (½-cup) servings

NUTRITION AT A GLANCE

Per serving: 230 calories, 6 g fat, 1 g saturated fat, 16 g protein, 32 g carbohydrate, 6 g dietary fiber, 105 mg sodium

MY SOUTH BEACH DIET

I'm now confident enough to pursue my dreams.

It's hard to believe that an active bodybuilder would need to lose weight, but at 5 feet 3 inches and 176 pounds, no one could see the muscle I worked so hard to achieve. I would spend almost 2 hours at the gym, 5 days a week—even the professional bodybuilders would comment on my "intensity" of training. However, I was always 15 to 30 (or more!) pounds overweight, and the layer of fat over all that muscle made me look stocky, not built.

I just assumed that my weight was genetic—obesity runs in my family. I remember remarking to my wife a month before starting the South Beach Diet, "I guess this is just as good as my body gets, given my genetics."

I first heard about the South Beach Diet from my wife. She had gone to her ob-gyn and mentioned that she wanted to lose some weight. Her doctor suggested the South Beach Diet. Like many people, we decided to give it a go on the first of the year—but I never would have guessed the results! At first, portion size (particularly for meat) was daunting, and it was difficult to cut out the processed "bad" carbs and fruit during Phase 1, but I was committed to this lifestyle. Many things surprised me while I reworked my eating habits: The South Beach recipes were delicious, I could snack between meals, and I ate enough so that I never felt hungry. This definitely was not like any other diet I had heard about in the past.

Now I'm down 30 pounds, and the results of my intense workouts can clearly be seen. That six-pack of abdominal muscles finally shows! I find myself enjoying great recipes like Turkey Parmesan, Beef Burritos, and Warm Artichoke Dip. Now that I am at my target weight, when we go out to dinner, I may have a dinner roll as an indulgence, maybe even clam chowder, but I find it's really easy to order within the guidelines of the South Beach Diet. And, of course, I'm right back to the lifestyle the next day.

I've received so many compliments due to my weight loss. From "You look 10 years younger" to my wife's boss saying, "Who is that buff guy?" before she recognized me. The best part: I now have the self-esteem to pursue personal training—something I have wanted to do for a long time but did not have the confidence when I was 30 pounds heavier. My wife is proud of me, and I am definitely proud of myself. Thank you, South Beach!

—*JOE H., PORT ST. LUCIE, FLORIDA*

Classic Ratatouille

PREP TIME: 10 minutes   **COOK TIME:** 25 minutes

A savory mix of cooked summer squash, eggplant, and tomatoes, this versatile Southern French dish is as easy to prepare as it is versatile: Serve it hot, cold, or at room temperature with chicken, fish, or meat—or as a salad on its own. The juicier and riper the tomatoes, the fuller the flavor of the dish.

Make a double batch over the weekend and enjoy it throughout the week.

2 tablespoons extra-virgin olive oil, divided

1 (¾-pound) eggplant, cut into ½-inch cubes

1 medium onion, roughly chopped

3 garlic cloves, minced

1 red bell pepper, cut into ½-inch pieces

2 medium zucchini, cut into ½-inch pieces

1 large tomato, cut into ½-inch pieces

1 tablespoon dried basil

Salt and freshly ground black pepper

Heat 1 tablespoon of the oil in a large, heavy-bottomed saucepan over medium heat. Add eggplant and a pinch of salt; cook, stirring occasionally, until lightly browned, about 5 minutes. Remove from the pan and set aside.

Add remaining oil to the same saucepan; raise heat to medium-high. Add onion and cook, stirring occasionally, until softened, about 3 minutes; add garlic and cook 1 minute more.

Add bell pepper and zucchini; cook until beginning to soften, about 5 minutes. Add tomato, basil, and a pinch of salt and pepper; cook 5 minutes more.

Return eggplant to the pan, reduce heat to low, cover, and cook, stirring occasionally, until vegetables are softened, about 5 minutes; season with salt and pepper to taste. Refrigerate, up to 3 days, until ready to eat.

Makes 4 (1-cup) servings

NUTRITION AT A GLANCE

Per serving: 130 calories, 8 g fat, 1 g saturated fat, 3 g protein, 16 g carbohydrate, 6 g dietary fiber, 90 mg sodium

Celery Root and Turnip Mash

PREP TIME: 10 minutes   **COOK TIME:** 30 minutes

Celery root (sometimes called celeriac) and turnip may not be common sightings in your kitchen, but once you try this creamy, delicious alternative to plain old mashed potatoes, you're likely to become hooked! Look for fresh, firm, unblemished vegetables and keep them stored in a cool dry place; the fresher they are, the faster they'll cook.

- 1 pound celery root, peeled and cut into ½-inch pieces
- 1 pound turnips, peeled and cut into ½-inch pieces
- ⅓ cup fat-free half-and-half
- 2 tablespoons trans-fat-free margarine
- Salt and freshly ground black pepper

Place celery root and turnips in a large saucepan, cover with salted cold water, and bring to a low boil; cook until very tender, about 25 minutes. Drain, transfer to a food processor, add half-and-half and margarine, and blend until smooth. Season with salt and pepper to taste and serve.

Makes 6 (½-cup) servings

NUTRITION AT A GLANCE

Per serving: 90 calories, 3.5 g fat, 1 g saturated fat, 2 g protein, 13 g carbohydrate, 3 g dietary fiber, 210 mg sodium

Spinach with Garlic and Pine Nuts

PREP TIME: 10 minutes   **COOK TIME:** 8 minutes

When shopping for spinach, choose the thicker, shinier spinach leaves for sautéing. The flat, more delicate spinach is better for eating raw.

1 pound spinach leaves, tough stems removed (7 to 8 cups loosely packed)

1 tablespoon extra-virgin olive oil

2 tablespoons pine nuts

2 garlic cloves, sliced

Salt and freshly ground black pepper

Wash spinach and spin dry, leaving some droplets of water on leaves.

Heat oil in a large skillet over medium heat. Add pine nuts and cook, stirring frequently, until lightly golden, about 3 minutes. Add garlic and cook 1 minute more.

Add spinach to the pan, in batches if necessary, and sauté until starting to wilt, 30 seconds. Cook, stirring and tossing frequently until all spinach is wilted and liquid is absorbed, about 3 minutes. Season with salt and pepper and serve.

Makes 4 (¾-cup) servings

NUTRITION AT A GLANCE

Per serving: 90 calories, 7 g fat, 1 g saturated fat, 4 g protein, 5 g carbohydrate, 3 g dietary fiber, 160 mg sodium

South Beach Cole Slaw

PREP TIME: 20 minutes

Who can get through a summer without this crisp and refreshing seasonal favorite? If you have a food processor, use it for quick cabbage shredding.

> 1 cup mayonnaise
>
> 3 tablespoons Dijon mustard
>
> 3 tablespoons cider vinegar
>
> 1½ teaspoons celery seed
>
> 1 teaspoon granular sugar substitute
>
> 1 small (1- to 1½-pound) head green cabbage, shredded (4 cups)
>
> 1 small (1- to 1½-pound) head red cabbage, shredded (4 cups)
>
> Salt and freshly ground black pepper

Whisk together mayonnaise, mustard, vinegar, celery seed, and sugar substitute. Add cabbage and toss to combine. Season to taste with salt and pepper and refrigerate until ready to serve.

Makes 16 (½-cup) servings

NUTRITION AT A GLANCE

Per serving: 110 calories, 11 g fat, 1.5 g saturated fat, 1 g protein, 3 g carbohydrate, 0 g dietary fiber, 150 mg sodium

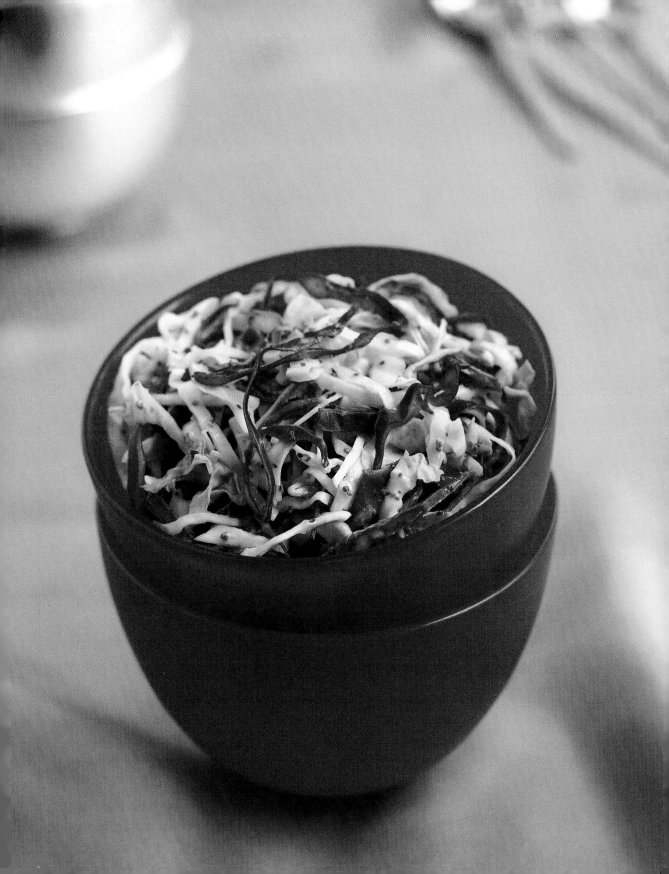

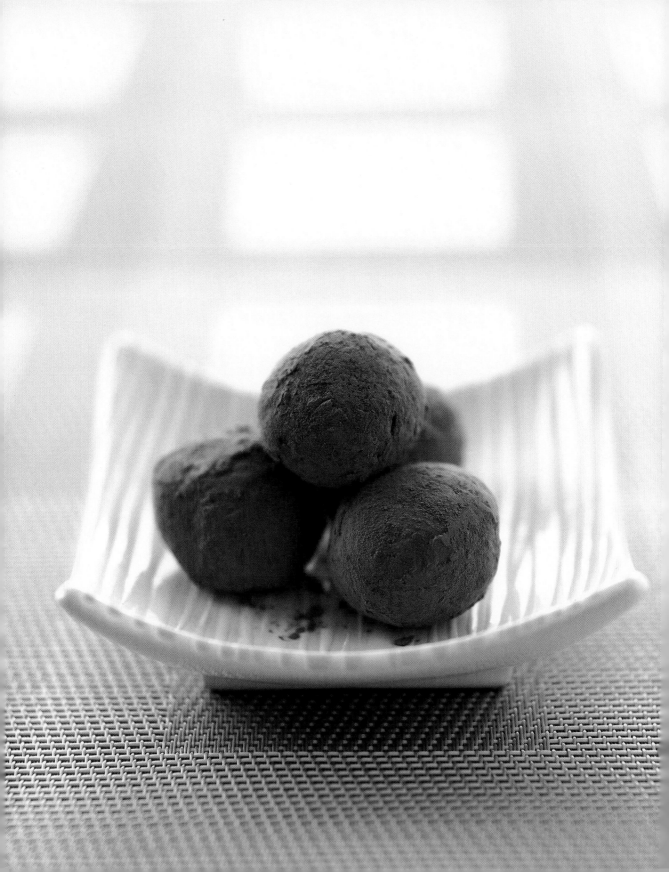

DESSERTS

In moderation and with the right ingredients, dessert not only satisfies your sweet tooth, it can actually provide nutrients. In our Green Tea Truffles, for example, bittersweet chocolate and green tea offer valuable antioxidants and flavanoids.

And since dessert should be fun, we've included easy Peanut Butter and Jelly Cookies and Mexican-Style Chocolate Bananas, and more. And for those occasions that call for a dressed-up end to the meal, there's a pear tart made with a crisp, paper-thin crust and an elegant cherry spoon sweet with yogurt.

We've also included a handful of flourless treats, like Melon Slush; Mini Cocoa Swirl Cheesecakes; Rice Pudding flavored with orange zest, almonds, and cinnamon; and Raspberry-Chocolate Cakes.

◄ *Green Tea Truffles (page 442)*

Green Tea Truffles

PREP TIME: 30 minutes

Both green tea and dark chocolate are packed with antioxidants, making this decadent treat much healthier (when eaten in moderation) than one you might buy in a chocolate shop. Once you master this easy recipe, you can try any of your favorite teas, such as Earl Gray, in place of green.

- ¾ cup fat-free half-and-half
- 4 decaffeinated green tea bags
- ½ pound bittersweet chocolate (preferably 65 percent cocoa), finely chopped
- ¼ cup unsweetened cocoa powder

Heat half-and-half in a small saucepan over medium heat. When it comes to a simmer, remove from heat and add tea bags; allow tea to steep 5 minutes.

Gently squeeze bags over half-and-half to extract extra flavor and discard. Return to a simmer and pour over chopped chocolate in a medium bowl. Stir to combine. Place bowl in freezer until set, about 10 minutes, removing and stirring every 2 minutes. Chocolate is ready to roll into truffles when it is no longer a pudding-like consistency and is starting to harden.

Scoop out about 2 teaspoons chocolate mixture and roll in the palms of your hands to form a 1-inch ball. Repeat with remaining chocolate. Place cocoa powder in a shallow dish. Roll balls in the cocoa powder to coat.

Shake off any excess cocoa powder (you will have 2 tablespoons remaining). Serve or store in an airtight container in the refrigerator for up to 2 weeks.

Makes 16 (2-piece) servings

NUTRITION AT A GLANCE

Per serving: 90 calories, 5 g fat, 3 g saturated fat, 1 g protein, 9 g carbohydrate, 1 g dietary fiber, 15 mg sodium

Mexican-Style Chocolate Bananas

PREP TIME: 10 minutes   **COOK TIME:** 2 minutes
CHILL TIME: 15 minutes

Cinnamon—which lends a Mexican flair—plus a little bit of chocolate are all you need to get big flavor out of these small bites. Serve them while the chocolate is still warm or chill them, allowing the chocolate to harden to a delectable crunch.

- ⅓ cup bittersweet chocolate chips
- ¼ teaspoon ground cinnamon
- 2 medium bananas, peeled and cut into 8 pieces each

Heat chocolate in a small skillet over low heat until melted, about 2 minutes. Add cinnamon and stir to combine.

Holding 1 piece of banana by the end, dip it into the chocolate mixture to coat the other end. Place it, chocolate end up, on a clean plate. Repeat with remaining banana pieces, coating the pointed ends of the four "tip" pieces (gently reheat chocolate if necessary). Serve or place in the refrigerator until chocolate hardens, about 15 minutes.

Makes 4 (4-piece) servings

NUTRITION AT A GLANCE

Per serving: 130 calories, 5 g fat, 2.5 g saturated fat, 1 g protein, 23 g carbohydrate, 2 g dietary fiber, 0 mg sodium

Mini Cocoa Swirl Cheesecakes

PREP TIME: 10 minutes

COOK TIME: 20 minutes   **CHILL TIME:** 2 hours

Ricotta cheese mixed with reduced-fat cream cheese and cocoa makes a rich and creamy chocolatey dessert. Muffin tins produce individual servings, perfect for family or a party. Prep and bake times are quick, but you'll want to prepare this dessert in advance, so you can allow it to chill in the refrigerator before serving.

6 ounces reduced-fat cream cheese, at room temperature

½ cup part-skim ricotta cheese

2 tablespoons granular sugar substitute

1 large egg

1 large egg yolk

½ teaspoon vanilla extract

1½ teaspoons unsweetened cocoa powder, sifted

Heat oven to 350°F. Line 6 muffin cups with paper or foil liners.

Blend cream cheese and ricotta in a food processor until creamy. Add sugar substitute, egg, egg yolk, and vanilla; process until smooth.

Divide 1 cup of the batter among the muffin cups. Add cocoa powder to the remaining batter and combine. Drop a heaping tablespoon of the cocoa batter into each muffin cup and gently fold to form a swirl.

Place the muffin tin in a large roasting pan and fill the pan with hot water to reach halfway up the tin. Bake until the cakes are puffed and set, 18 to 20 minutes. Remove from the water and cool at room temperature. Refrigerate until chilled, about 2 hours.

Makes 6 servings

NUTRITION AT A GLANCE

Per serving: 130 calories, 8 g fat, 4.5 g saturated fat, 7 g protein, 7 g carbohydrate, 0 g dietary fiber, 125 mg sodium

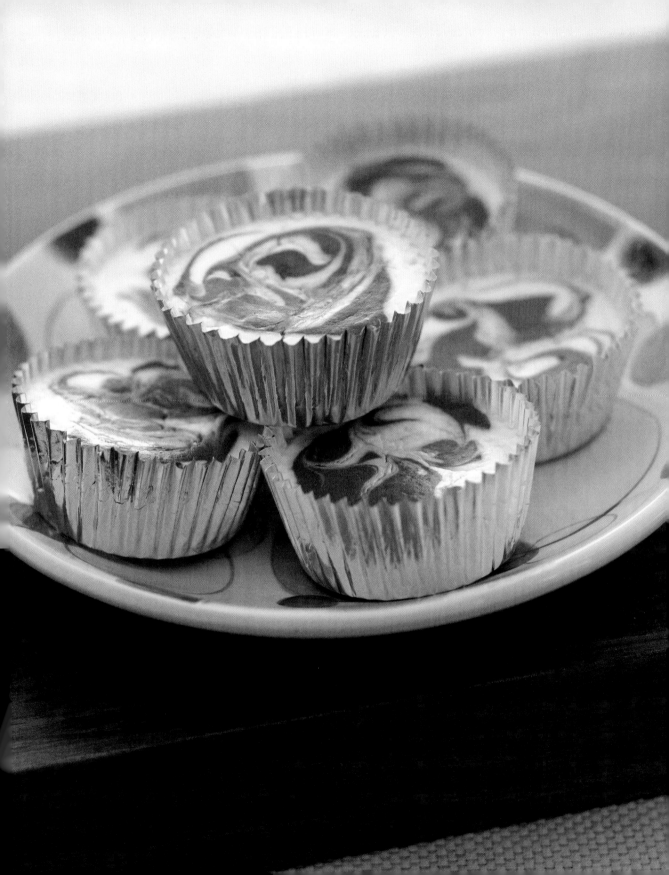

Chocolate Pudding

PREP TIME: 5 minutes **COOK TIME:** 10 minutes
CHILL TIME: 3 hours

There's no contest when it comes to chocolate pudding—it's a creamy indulgence we can all afford to enjoy from time to time, especially when eating the South Beach version! Again, prep and cook times are quick, but the pudding does need to be chilled before serving.

> 2 cups fat-free half-and-half, divided
>
> 1 packet unflavored gelatin
>
> ¼ cup granular sugar substitute
>
> ⅓ cup unsweetened cocoa powder
>
> Pinch salt
>
> 3 tablespoons bittersweet chocolate chips
>
> ½ teaspoon vanilla extract

Pour ½ cup of the half-and-half into a small bowl. Sprinkle gelatin on top and set aside until softened, about 5 minutes.

Meanwhile, combine sugar substitute, cocoa powder, and salt in a medium saucepan; whisk in the remaining half-and-half. Bring cocoa mixture to a boil over medium heat, whisking constantly. Remove from heat, add chocolate chips, and let stand for 1 minute. Whisk until smooth.

Add gelatin mixture to cocoa mixture and stir until dissolved. Stir in vanilla and divide among 4 serving cups. Cover each cup with plastic wrap and chill in the coldest part of the refrigerator until firm, about 3 hours or overnight.

Makes 4 (1/2-cup) servings

NUTRITION AT A GLANCE

Per serving: 140 calories, 5 g fat, 3 g saturated fat, 6 g protein, 21 g carbohydrate, 3 g dietary fiber, 250 mg sodium

Thin and Crispy Pear Tart

PREP TIME: 15 minutes   **COOK TIME:** 22 minutes

This tart is simple yet elegant. Serve it warm with a dollop of crème fraîche or plain fat-free or low-fat yogurt.

- 1 tablespoon fresh lemon juice
- 1 tablespoon granular sugar substitute
- ⅛ teaspoon ground cinnamon
- ½ teaspoon almond extract
- 2 medium Bosc pears, sliced ⅛ inch thick
- 6 (13 by 18-inch) sheets frozen whole-wheat phyllo dough, thawed

  Butter-flavored cooking spray

Heat oven to 375°F. Combine lemon juice, sugar substitute, cinnamon, and almond extract in a medium bowl. Add pears and stir to coat.

Line a baking sheet with parchment paper. Working quickly, lay 1 phyllo sheet on the baking sheet, coat lightly with cooking spray, fold in half widthwise, and lightly coat with spray again. Repeat with remaining sheets, piling sheets in a single stack as you go.

Fold edges in ¼ inch on each side. Lay pear slices on top of phyllo in a single layer. Bake until pears are tender and crust is golden, about 22 minutes. Serve warm.

Makes 4 servings

NUTRITION AT A GLANCE

Per serving: 130 calories, 2 g fat, 0 g saturated fat, 2 g protein, 27 g carbohydrate, 3 g dietary fiber, 140 mg sodium

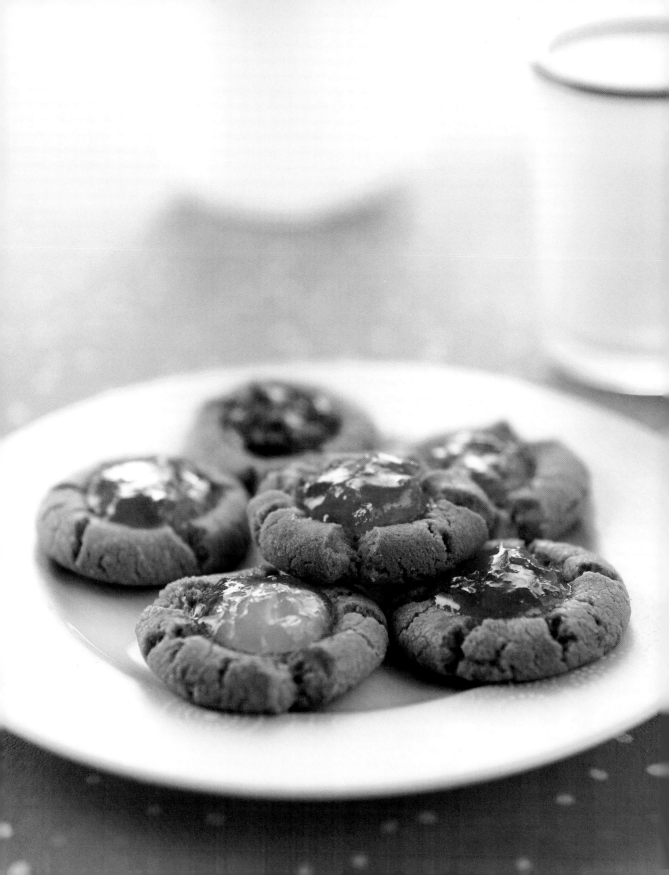

Peanut Butter and Jelly Cookies

PREP TIME: 15 minutes   **COOK TIME:** 14 minutes

Who would believe you can get such a delectable cookie out of such a simple process and with so few ingredients? (That's right, there's no flour!) The not-too-sweet, deep nutty flavor—topped with a touch of fruit—is perfect for kids young and old. These cookies are so good that I need to remind you to limit yourself to one serving!

- ¾ cup granular sugar substitute
- 1 large egg
- 1 teaspoon vanilla extract
- 1 cup creamy trans-fat-free peanut butter
- 1 teaspoon baking soda
- ¼ cup sugar-free jam, any flavor

Heat oven to 350°F. Line a baking sheet with parchment paper.

Mix sugar substitute, egg, and vanilla together with an electric mixer on low for 3 minutes. Add peanut butter and baking soda. Mix on medium until dough comes together, about 30 seconds.

Form dough into 24 (2-teaspoon) balls and place on baking sheet 1 inch apart. Gently press your thumb into the center of each to make an indentation. Fill each indentation with ½ teaspoon jam.

Bake until lightly browned on the bottom, 12 to 14 minutes. Transfer to a wire rack to cool completely.

Makes 12 (2-piece) servings

NUTRITION AT A GLANCE

Per serving: 140 calories, 11 g fat, 2.5 g saturated fat, 6 g protein, 7 g carbohydrate, 1 g dietary fiber, 210 mg sodium

Nutty Brownies

PREP TIME: 10 minutes   **COOK TIME:** 25 minutes

Nuts mixed with chocolate is a classic combination and, in these moist brownies, a pure delight! Brownies freeze well in resealable freezer bags, so you can easily save some for a later date.

- ¾ cup walnuts
- ¾ cup granular sugar substitute
- ¼ cup unsweetened cocoa powder
- ½ teaspoon baking powder
- ½ teaspoon salt
- 3 large eggs, lightly beaten
- ½ cup reduced-fat sour cream
- ¼ cup extra-virgin olive oil
- 2 teaspoons vanilla extract
- ½ cup bittersweet chocolate chips

Heat oven to 350°F. Lightly coat an 8- by 8-inch baking pan with cooking spray.

Pulse walnuts in a food processor until finely chopped. Place in a large mixing bowl; add sugar substitute, cocoa powder, baking powder, and salt. Whisk to combine.

Whisk together eggs, sour cream, oil, and vanilla. Make a well in dry ingredients and whisk wet into dry to combine.

Heat chocolate chips in a small saucepan over medium-low heat, whisking constantly to melt, about 1 minute. Whisk into batter.

Pour batter into pan and bake until a toothpick inserted in the center comes out clean, 20 to 25 minutes. Cool completely, cut into 16 squares, and serve.

Makes 16 servings

NUTRITION AT A GLANCE

Per serving: 130 calories, 11 g fat, 2.5 g saturated fat, 3 g protein, 6 g carbohydrate, 1 g dietary fiber, 100 mg sodium

Coconut Wafers

PREP TIME: 10 minutes   **COOK TIME:** 24 minutes

Serve these crispy cookies atop a bowl of ripe fresh berries.

    2 large egg whites
    ⅛ teaspoon salt
    2 tablespoons granular sugar substitute
    2 tablespoons sugar
    ½ teaspoon vanilla extract
    2 tablespoons whole-wheat flour
    ¾ cup unsweetened shredded coconut
    2 tablespoons trans-fat-free margarine, melted

Heat oven to 350°F. Line a baking pan with foil and lightly coat with cooking spray.

Whisk egg whites, salt, sugar substitute, sugar, and vanilla in a medium bowl until light and foamy, about 2 minutes. Sift in flour and stir to combine. Stir in coconut. Slowly whisk in margarine until incorporated.

Drop 6 (2-teaspoon) balls of batter onto pan. Using a butter knife, spread each ball into a 3-inch disk. Bake until the edges are golden, about 12 minutes. Transfer to a wire rack to cool completely. Repeat with the remaining batter. Store in an airtight container for up to 1 week.

Makes 6 (2-piece) servings

NUTRITION AT A GLANCE

Per serving: 150 calories, 11 g fat, 8 g saturated fat, 2 g protein, 12 g carbohydrate, 2 g dietary fiber, 100 mg sodium

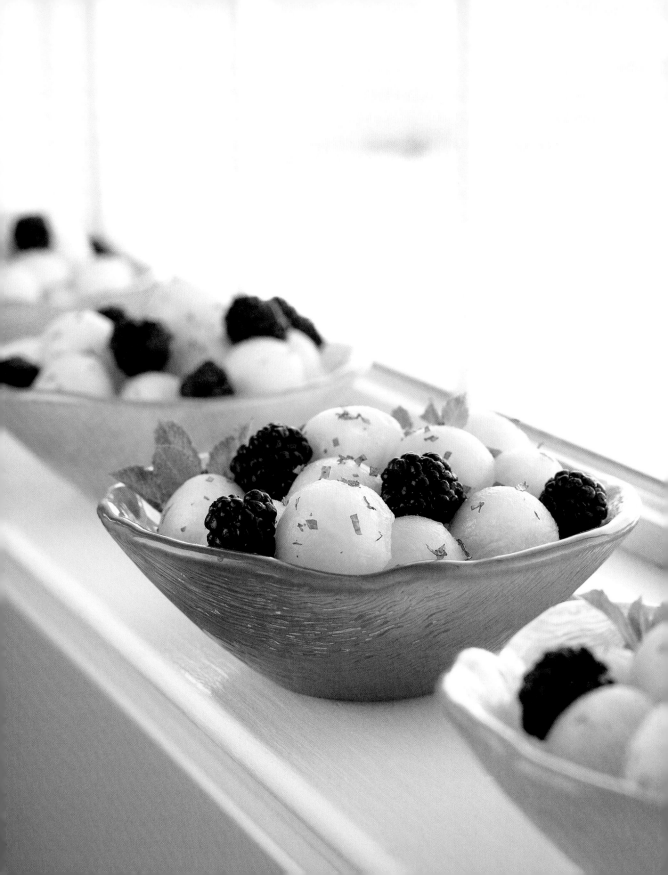

Fruit Salad with Lime and Mint

PREP TIME: 10 minutes

*Serve this refreshing and very pretty dessert as is or with a
dollop of plain fat-free or low-fat yogurt.*

3 cups honeydew melon balls

2 cups blueberries, blackberries, or a mix

1 heaping tablespoon chopped fresh mint

1 tablespoon fresh lime juice

Place melon balls, berries, mint, and lime juice in a
mixing bowl and toss to combine. Serve cold in bowls
or martini glasses.

Makes 4 (1¼-cup) servings

NUTRITION AT A GLANCE

Per serving: 90 calories, 0 g fat, 0 g saturated fat, 1 g protein,
23 g carbohydrate, 3 g dietary fiber, 25 mg sodium

Rice Pudding

PREP TIME: 15 minutes   **COOK TIME:** 10 minutes

Rice pudding fans love the dessert's tender, creamy texture. On the South Beach Diet, you can have your pudding and get your nutrients too, as brown rice is high in B vitamins and minerals.

2 cups cooked whole-grain, quick-cooking brown rice (page 14)

1 cup fat-free half-and-half

2 tablespoons granular sugar substitute

1 tablespoon grated orange zest

1 teaspoon vanilla extract

1 tablespoon sliced almonds (optional)

Ground cinnamon (optional)

Salt

Bring rice, half-and-half, sugar substitute, orange zest, vanilla, and a pinch of salt to a low boil in a medium saucepan over medium heat. Reduce to a low simmer and cook, stirring frequently, until liquid is absorbed, 6 to 8 minutes. Top with almonds and/or a pinch of cinnamon, if using, and serve hot.

Makes 4 (¹/₂-cup) servings

NUTRITION AT A GLANCE

Per serving: 170 calories, 1.5 g fat, ½ g saturated fat, 4 g protein, 33 g carbohydrate, 2 g dietary fiber, 160 mg sodium

Flourless Chocolate-Raspberry Cakes

PREP TIME: 15 minutes   **COOK TIME:** 15 minutes

These adorable mini cakes are rich, moist, and very chocolatey—and they freeze well, making it easy to get a head start on a party or to just enjoy a cake from time to time without having to bake a whole batch. You can replace half of the sugar substitute with granulated sugar, if you'd like; baking time may increase by a few minutes.

¾ cup bittersweet chocolate chips

½ cup trans-fat-free margarine

½ cup granular sugar substitute

½ cup unsweetened cocoa powder, sifted

3 large eggs

½ cup raspberries

Position rack in middle of oven and heat to 375°F. Line a muffin tin with paper or foil liners.

Heat chocolate and margarine in a heavy saucepan over low heat until melted, about 4 minutes; stir to combine and remove from heat.

Mix sugar substitute and cocoa powder in a medium mixing bowl; add eggs and whisk until combined. Whisk in chocolate mixture.

Scoop batter into the tin (about 2½ tablespoons per muffin cup), gently press 3 raspberries halfway into each cake, and place the pan on a baking sheet. Bake, turning once halfway through, until a thin crust forms on top, 12 to 15 minutes. Cool on a wire rack and serve.

Makes 12 servings

NUTRITION AT A GLANCE

Per serving: 140 calories, 11 g fat, 4 g saturated fat, 3 g protein, 11 g carbohydrate, 2 g dietary fiber, 80 mg sodium

Cherry Spoon Sweet with Yogurt

PREP TIME: 5 minutes   **COOK TIME: 10 minutes**

This easy-to-make fresh fruit jam turns yogurt into a special dessert. Leftover "spoon sweet" will keep, refrigerated, for up to 10 days and can double as a spread for whole-grain toast or as a topping for reduced-fat cottage cheese.

- 1 (16-ounce) package unsweetened bing cherries
- 1 teaspoon grated lemon zest
- 2 tablespoons granular sugar substitute
- 24 ounces plain fat-free or low-fat yogurt

Bring cherries, lemon zest, and sugar substitute to a simmer in a small saucepan over medium-low heat. Cook, stirring occasionally, until cherries have softened, about 5 minutes. Remove from heat and cool slightly.

Divide yogurt among 4 serving dishes. Top each serving with ¼ cup of the cherries and serve.

Makes 4 (1-cup) servings

NUTRITION AT A GLANCE

Per serving: 200 calories, 4 g fat, 1.5 g saturated fat, 10 g protein, 34 g carbohydrate, 2 g dietary fiber, 115 mg sodium

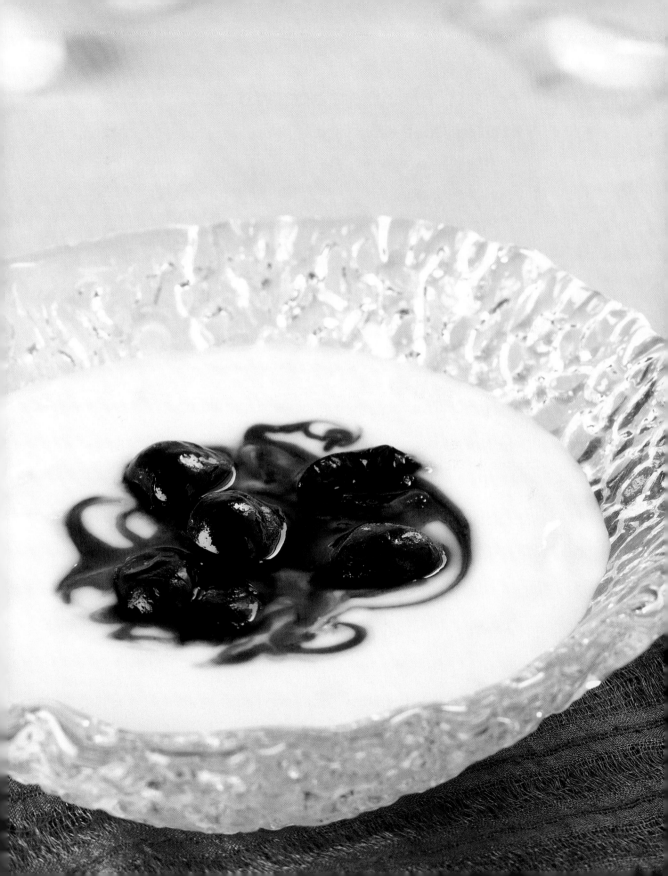

Creamy Dreamy Strawberry Vanilla Shake

PREP TIME: 5 minutes

Frozen strawberries work like ice cubes to thicken and chill this irresistibly creamy shake. Since the berries are available year-round, you can enjoy it anytime.

1 cup plain fat-free or low-fat yogurt

1 cup 1 percent milk

2 cups frozen strawberries

1 teaspoon vanilla extract

Purée yogurt, milk, strawberries, and vanilla in a blender until smooth. Serve cold.

Makes 4 (1-cup) servings

NUTRITION AT A GLANCE

Per serving: 90 calories, 1.5 g fat, 1 g saturated fat, 6 g protein, 14 g carbohydrate, 1 g dietary fiber, 75 mg sodium

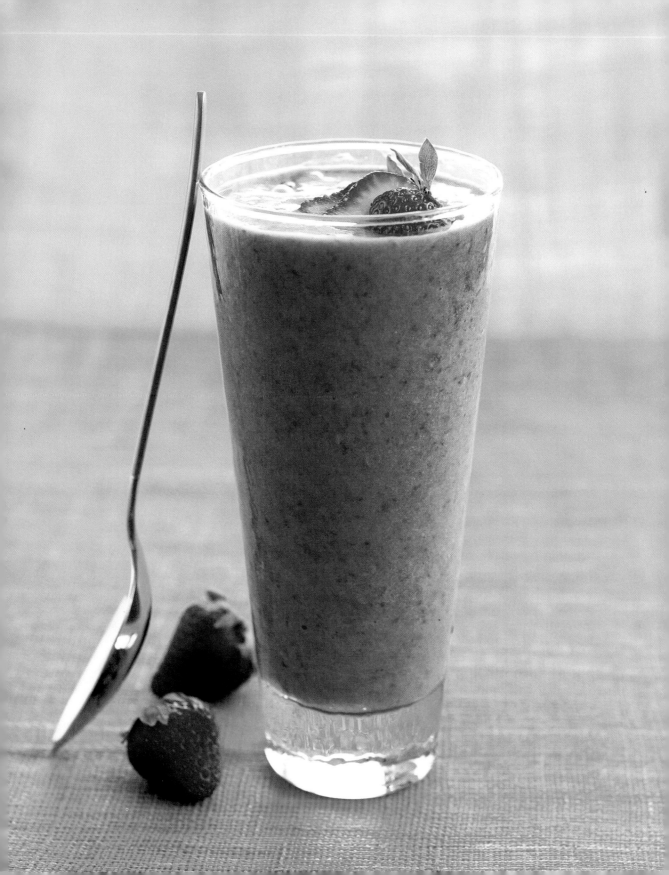

Orange Poppy Seed Cupcakes

PREP TIME: 15 minutes   **COOK TIME:** 25 minutes

Light as a feather, these delicious cakes are as pretty as they are moist. You can freeze them if you'd like—freeze before icing, defrost fully, and put the icing on just before serving. Purchase separated egg whites, so you don't have to spend time separating eggs.

- 12 large egg whites, at room temperature (¾ cup)
- 1¼ teaspoons cream of tartar
- ¼ teaspoon salt
- 1 teaspoon vanilla extract
- ½ teaspoon orange extract, plus extra for topping
- ¾ cup granular sugar substitute
- ¾ cup whole-grain pastry flour
- 1 tablespoon poppy seeds
- 1 cup light or fat-free whipped topping

Heat oven to 350°F. Line 18 standard muffin cups with paper liners.

Combine egg whites, cream of tartar, and salt in a large metal mixing bowl. Whisk until soft peaks form. Add vanilla and orange extracts. Gradually add sugar substitute, beating whites until stiff.

Sift one-third of the flour over egg whites and fold with a rubber spatula to gently but fully combine. Repeat with remaining flour until all of the flour is incorporated, then add poppy seeds.

Fill muffin cups with mixture, filling them just over the top of each cup (cupcakes will not rise while cooking). Bake, turning once, until tops are golden and dry and a toothpick inserted in the center comes out clean, 20 to 25 minutes. Cool completely.

Mix whipped topping with 3 or 4 drops orange extract to make frosting. Place a dollop of whipped topping on each cupcake and serve.

Makes 18 servings

NUTRITION AT A GLANCE

Per serving: 40 calories, 1 g fat, 0 g saturated fat, 3 g protein, 5 g carbohydrate, 0 g dietary fiber, 70 mg sodium

Flourless Fig and Almond Bites

PREP TIME: 5 minutes   **COOK TIME: 25 minutes**

Here's a not-too-sweet dessert that's also a perfect snack with a cup of midday coffee or tea. But don't be fooled by the lack of flour, butter, and sugar in these rich cookies—they simply don't need any. Figs lend natural sweetness, and almond meal offers body and a buttery rich flavor. Almond meal, which is just ground almonds, can be found in most health food stores, or you can grind your own.

- 2 cups almond meal (or finely ground almonds)
- 1 cup (6 ounces) soft dried figs, hard tips removed and discarded
- 2 teaspoons finely grated orange zest
- 1 teaspoon vanilla extract
- ½ teaspoon salt

Position rack in upper third of oven and heat to 325°F. Lightly coat a baking sheet with cooking spray or line with parchment paper.

Blend almond meal, figs, orange zest, vanilla, and salt in a food processor until mixture resembles coarse meal and has the texture of wet sand, about 1 minute.

Form dough into 30 (2-teaspoon) slightly flattened balls and place on baking sheet ½ inch apart (cookies will not spread during baking).

Bake until bottoms of cookies are lightly browned, 12 to 15 minutes, turning pan once halfway through. Cool and serve.

Makes 15 (2-piece) servings

NUTRITION AT A GLANCE

Per serving: 160 calories, 10 g fat, 1 g saturated fat, 5 g protein, 17 g carbohydrate, 4 g dietary fiber, 30 mg sodium

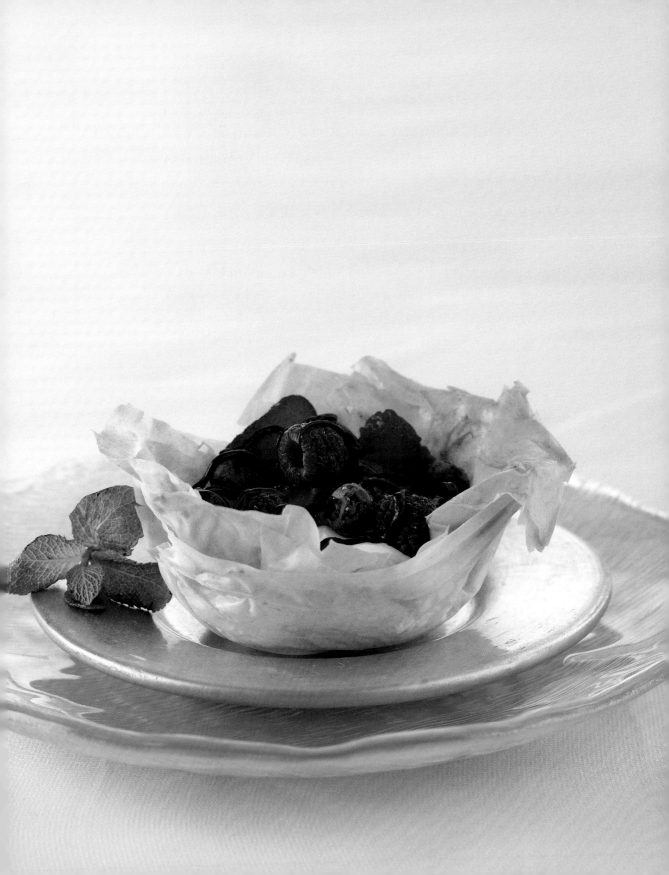

Chocolate Berry Cups

PREP TIME: 10 minutes   **COOK TIME:** 15 minutes

Fruit and chocolate lovers will appreciate this tasty treat. The cups can be made ahead and stored in an airtight container for up to 3 days, making this an easy holiday or party dessert—assemble the rest just before serving. Look for whole-wheat phyllo in supermarkets and health food stores.

- 1 cup mixed berries (blueberries, raspberries, and/or sliced strawberries)
- 1 tablespoon granular sugar substitute
- 2 (13- by 18-inch) sheets frozen whole-wheat phyllo dough, thawed
- 1½ tablespoons trans-fat-free margarine, melted
- 1 ounce bittersweet chocolate, chopped
- ¼ cup part-skim ricotta or South Beach Ricotta Crème

Heat oven to 350°F.

Combine berries with sugar substitute. Spread 1 phyllo sheet out on a clean work surface. Lightly brush with margarine. Lay second sheet on top of first; brush with margarine. Fold sheets in half widthwise. Brush top side with more margarine.

Cut dough in half lengthwise, then again widthwise to create 4 equal pieces. Carefully fit each piece into a nonstick muffin pan to create a cup. Bake the cups until golden brown, about 15 minutes. Set aside to cool.

When you are ready to assemble cups, place chocolate in a resealable plastic bag. Heat, unsealed, in the microwave at 30-second intervals until melted, about 2 minutes. Fill each phyllo cup with 1 tablespoon ricotta and ¼ cup berries. Cut a tiny corner off one bottom corner of the plastic bag with scissors; press chocolate toward the corner and drizzle over berries.

Makes 4 servings

NUTRITION AT A GLANCE

Per serving: 160 calories, 10 g fat, 5 g saturated fat, 2 g protein, 16 g carbohydrate, 3 g dietary fiber, 80 mg sodium

Spiced Chocolate Nut Clusters

PREP TIME: 5 minutes   **FREEZE TIME:** 10 minutes

Here's a nutty, crunchy dessert that comes together in just 15 minutes. Macadamia nuts, known as a "gourmet, dessert variety," have a delicious creamy, rich texture, but you can substitute any favorite nut in this recipe. Though nuts are healthy, they are also high in fat, so remember to stick to two clusters per portion.

⅓ cup bittersweet chocolate chips

¼ cup fat-free half-and-half

½ teaspoon ground cinnamon

½ teaspoon vanilla extract

1 cup whole macadamia nuts, chopped

Line a baking sheet with parchment paper. Warm chocolate, half-and-half, and cinnamon in a medium saucepan over medium-low heat, stirring constantly, until chocolate is melted, about 2 minutes.

Remove from heat, add vanilla, and stir to combine. Add nuts and stir to coat. Drop 12 (1-tablespoon) clusters onto the baking sheet. Freeze for 10 minutes to set. Store in the refrigerator.

Makes 6 (2-piece) servings

NUTRITION AT A GLANCE

Per serving: 210 calories, 21 g fat, 5 g saturated fat, 3 g protein, 9 g carbohydrate, 2 g dietary fiber, 15 mg sodium

Chocolate-Walnut Macaroons

PREP TIME: 15 minutes   **COOK TIME: 12 minutes**

These moist, chocolatey jewels brim with crunchy walnuts, the only nut that contains omega-3 fatty acids. Store shelled walnuts (and other nuts) in the refrigerator or freezer to keep them fresh over time.

  1 cup walnuts

  2 tablespoons granular sugar substitute

  2 tablespoons sugar

  2 tablespoons unsweetened cocoa powder

¼ teaspoon salt

  1 large egg white

½ teaspoon vanilla extract

Heat oven to 325°F. Line a baking sheet with parchment paper.

   Finely grind walnuts, sugar substitute, sugar, cocoa powder, and salt in a food processor. Add egg white and vanilla and pulse until mixture comes together.

Form dough into 12 (2-teaspoon) balls and place on baking sheet; gently press each ball to flatten. Bake until edges are firm to the touch, about 12 minutes. Cool on a wire rack and store in an airtight container for up to 5 days.

Makes 6 (2-piece) servings

NUTRITION AT A GLANCE

Per serving: 150 calories, 11 g fat, 1 g saturated fat, 4 g protein, 11 g carbohydrate, 2 g dietary fiber, 105 mg sodium

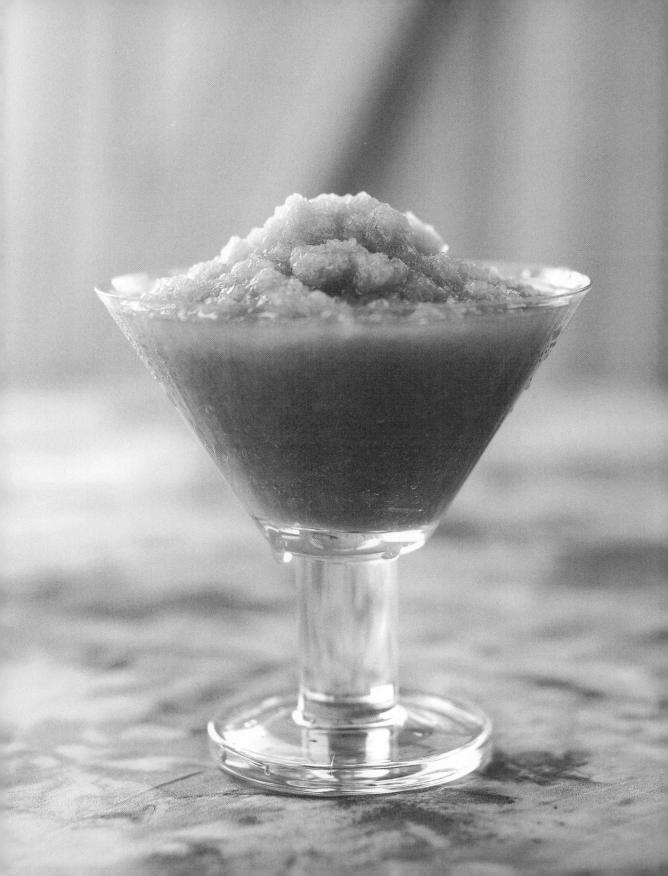

Melon Slush

PREP TIME: 5 minutes

This refreshing fruity slush comes together in minutes. Serve it in iced glasses for an extra-cool treat and keep cubed cantaloupe in the freezer so you can enjoy it anytime.

- 5 ice cubes
- 4 cups cubed cantaloupe
- 1½ teaspoons fresh lemon juice
- 1½ teaspoons granular sugar substitute

Place ice cubes in a blender and blend until just crushed. Add cantaloupe, lemon juice, and sugar substitute. Blend until combined, about 10 seconds. Serve immediately.

Makes 4 (1-cup) servings

NUTRITION AT A GLANCE

Per serving: 60 calories, 0 g fat, 0 g saturated fat, 1 g protein, 13 g carbohydrate, 1 g dietary fiber, 25 mg sodium

Lemon Olive Oil Cake

PREP TIME: 15 minutes   **COOK TIME:** 25 minutes

Made with extra-virgin olive oil instead of butter and whole-wheat instead of white flour, this cake is a healthful, yet deliciously moist and flavorful treat. The lively lemon flavor makes it perfect for serving on its own or with fresh fruit or plain low-fat yogurt.

1½	cups whole-grain pastry flour	¾	cup granular sugar substitute
½	teaspoon baking soda	½	cup 1 percent or fat-free buttermilk
½	teaspoon baking powder	½	cup extra-virgin olive oil
¼	teaspoon salt	2	teaspoons lemon extract
3	large eggs, separated	1	tablespoon grated lemon zest

Heat oven to 350°F. Lightly coat an 8-inch springform pan with cooking spray.

Whisk together flour, baking soda, baking powder, and salt in a large bowl; form a well in the center.

Beat egg whites with an electric mixer at high speed in a medium bowl until stiff peaks form, about 3 minutes.

Beat egg yolks, sugar substitute, buttermilk, oil, lemon extract, and lemon zest in a medium bowl at medium speed until smooth, about 1 minute.

Pour egg yolk mixture into the center of the dry ingredients; stir gently until just combined. Gently fold in half of the egg whites, then fold in the remaining egg whites.

Pour batter into pan and bake until edges are lightly browned and a toothpick inserted in the center of the cake comes out clean, 25 to 28 minutes. Let cool in the pan for 5 minutes; remove from the pan and transfer to a wire rack. Cut into wedges and serve warm or at room temperature.

Makes 10 servings

NUTRITION AT A GLANCE

Per serving: 190 calories, 13 g fat, 2 g saturated fat, 4 g protein, 13 g carbohydrate, 1 g dietary fiber, 180 mg sodium

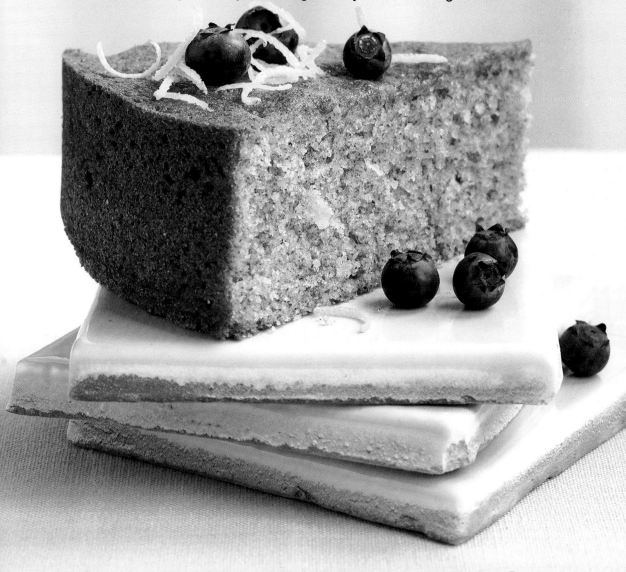

INDEX

Note: <u>Underscored</u> page references indicate boxed text.
Boldfaced page references indicate photographs.

Conversion Chart

These equivalents have been slightly rounded to make measuring easier.

VOLUME MEASUREMENTS

U.S.	Imperial	Metric
¼ tsp	–	1 ml
½ tsp	–	2 ml
1 tsp	–	5 ml
1 Tbsp	–	15 ml
2 Tbsp (1 oz)	1 fl oz	30 ml
¼ cup (2 oz)	2 fl oz	60 ml
⅓ cup (3 oz)	3 fl oz	80 ml
½ cup (4 oz)	4 fl oz	120 ml
⅔ cup (5 oz)	5 fl oz	160 ml
¾ cup (6 oz)	6 fl oz	180 ml
1 cup (8 oz)	8 fl oz	240 ml

WEIGHT MEASUREMENTS

U.S.	Metric
1 oz	30 g
2 oz	60 g
4 oz (¼ lb)	115 g
5 oz (⅓ lb)	145 g
6 oz	170 g
7 oz	200 g
8 oz (½ lb)	230 g
10 oz	285 g
12 oz (¾ lb)	340 g
14 oz	400 g
16 oz (1 lb)	455 g
2.2 lb	1 kg

LENGTH MEASUREMENTS

U.S.	Metric
¼"	0.6 cm
½"	1.25 cm
1"	2.5 cm
2"	5 cm
4"	11 cm
6"	15 cm
8"	20 cm
10"	25 cm
12" (1')	30 cm

PAN SIZES

U.S.	Metric
8" cake pan	20 × 4 cm sandwich or cake tin
9" cake pan	23 × 3.5 cm sandwich or cake tin
11" × 7" baking pan	28 × 18 cm baking tin
13" × 9" baking pan	32.5 × 23 cm baking tin
15" × 10" baking pan	38 × 25.5 cm baking tin (Swiss roll tin)
1½ qt baking dish	1.5 liter baking dish
2 qt baking dish	2 liter baking dish
2 qt rectangular baking dish	30 × 19 cm baking dish
9" pie plate	22 × 4 or 23 × 4 cm pie plate
7" or 8" springform pan	18 or 20 cm springform or loose-bottom cake tin
9" × 5" loaf pan	23 × 13 cm or 2 lb narrow loaf tin or pâté tin

TEMPERATURES

Fahrenheit	Centigrade	Gas
140°	60°	–
160°	70°	–
180°	80°	–
225°	105°	¼
250°	120°	½
275°	135°	1
300°	150°	2
325°	160°	3
350°	180°	4
375°	190°	5
400°	200°	6
425°	220°	7
450°	230°	8
475°	245°	9
500°	260°	–

LIKE WHAT YOU'VE SEEN?

If you enjoyed this large print edition of
The South Beach Diet Quick & Easy Cookbook, look for
other South Beach Diet books by Arthur Agatston, M.D.
which are also available in Random House Large Print.

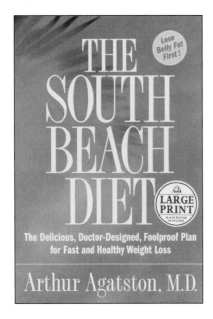

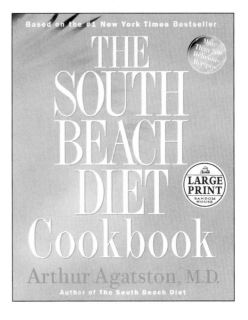

THE SOUTH BEACH DIET	**THE SOUTH BEACH**
(hardcover)	**DIET COOKBOOK**
0-375-43194-2	(hardcover)
$26.95/$39.95C	0-375-43343-0
	$25.95/$39.95C

Large print books are available wherever books
are sold and at many local libraries.

All prices are subject to change. Check with your
local retailer for current pricing and availability.
For more information on these and other large print titles,
visit www.randomlargeprint.com